John Staggs 11-2-77

Anatomical
Correlates
of Clinical
Electromyography

Dedicated to my Wife

Mildred Sylvia Goodgold

"Strength and dignity are her clothing"

Anatomical Correlates of Clinical Electromyography

Joseph Goodgold, M.D.

Director, Electrodiagnostic Service,
Institute of Rehabilitation Medicine
and University Hospital, New York
University Medical Center, and
Professor, New York University School
of Medicine, Department of
Rehabilitation Medicine

The Williams & Wilkins Company
Baltimore

Made in the United States of America

Reprinted 1975

Library of Congress Cataloging in Publication Data

Goodgold, Joseph.
Anatomical correlates of clinical electromyography.

   1. Electromyography. I. Title. [DNLM: 1. Electromyography. 2. Muscles—Anatomy and histology. WE141 G651a
1974]
RC77.5.G66   616.7'4'0754   74-5310
ISBN 0-683-03578-9

Composed and printed at the Waverly Press, Inc., Mt. Royal
and Guilford Aves., Baltimore, Md. 21202, U.S.A.

Foreword

Many have known the person who has a compulsive need to inform—witness the people who, when asked the time, respond with plans on how to make a clock!

Several years ago, Dr. Joseph Goodgold was visiting professor at Ohio State University for a continuing medical education course on electromyography. In one of the discussions, I pointed out the relative inaccessibility of the posterior tibial muscle to several participants who claimed it as a treasured muscle to explore electromyographically in lumbosacral radiculopathies. In point of fact, the electromyographer plunged the electrode into the ventromedial calf and pontifically announced he was "in the posterior tibial." Nonsense! He didn't know where he was! Dr. Goodgold agreed that my observation was quite correct.

Next Chapter

Through the mail came a beautiful line drawing of an anatomic cross section through the calf with an electromyographic needle electrode in place (and I framed it), showing clearly how to locate precisely the posterior tibial muscle.

This was the announcement that Dr. Goodgold was heavily into a text, detailed and exposite, showing the placement of intramuscular electromyographic electrodes. Now here it is—and beautifully done!

Logical sequential steps in the electromyographic examination first identify the electrical abnormality then carefully plot the distribution of the abnormalities. Here is where the indisputable knowledge of surface and neuromuscular anatomy is of primacy.

Whether the electrical abnormalities are in a root distribution, plexus, peripheral nerve or branch—or if the disease is generalized—all of these conclusions depend on accurate placement of the tip of the electromyographic needle and even more importantly, KNOWING where it is. During my 14 years of experience with the continuing education of clinical electromyographers, I have sampled their deficiencies by objective evaluation (i.e., multiple choice tests), and paradoxically the most fundamental knowledge necessary to perform electromyography is missing, i.e., basic anatomy.

All electromyographers—both student and experienced—please read! This treatise makes it A-B-C simple to speak with authority as the electromyographer uses electrodes and stimulators in the investigation of neuromuscular disease.

Ernest W. Johnson, M.D.
Professor and Chairman,
Department of Physical Medicine,
Ohio State University

Preface

This volume has been written with the purpose of bringing together certain essential anatomical information required by student and practitioner in the performance of clinical electromyography and nerve conduction studies. The text has been designed in modest proportions and is meant to be correlative rather than to replace standard texts and literature references. By no means is it an exhaustive anatomical book; in fact, information of relatively minor value in clinical assessment (i.e., kinesiological data) has been intentionally omitted. Actions of muscles are described to the limited extent of assistance in identification of the structure during electromyography; usually only the most important action is cited. The combination, however, of frontal and cross sectional views coupled with topography and landmark identification does seem to be relevant to the purpose of performance of concise electrophysiological examination. In most cases, the proper placement of the electrodes has been checked by bipolar stimulation after placing a second electrode in the muscle and using minute stimulating current to effect an isolated muscle response. This simple procedure of verification is highly recommended to the examiner when the least bit of question of accuracy exists. With regard to nomenclature, Latin and English names have been used interchangably as a matter of literary license. There is little doubt that recent medical graduates may find this text particularly useful because of the current severe restriction of the anatomy curriculum in our medical schools.

The author wishes to express his deep appreciation to the many colleagues at New York University and elsewhere, who reviewed, criticized and encouraged this work as it developed; special acknowledgment is made to my departmental Chairman at the New York University Medical Center, Howard A. Rusk, M.D., and to Ernest Johnson, M.D., Professor and Chairman, Department of Rehabilitation Medicine, Ohio State University who initially stimulated this undertaking.

The dedication and labors of my secretarial staff, particularly Mrs. Roberta Wailes, in preparation of this book is also worthy of special mention. Finally, my sincere thanks goes to Robert Wilson, Jr. Without his highly technical and professional skills as the illustrator who translated my hodgepodge of rough drawings and layouts into something meaningful, this book probably would not have progressed beyond a conceptional stage.

Contents

I HEAD AND NECK 1

   A. Muscles
      1. Facial
         a. Frontalis 2
         b. Orbicularis Oris 2
         c. Orbicularis Oculi 2
         d. Mentalis 2
      2. Masseter 2
      3. Posterior Auricular 4
      4. Tongue 6
      5. Sternocleidomastoid 8
      6. Levator Scapulae 8
      7. Cervical Paraspinal 10

II PECTORAL GIRDLE AND THORAX 13

   A. Muscles
      1. Trapezius 14
      2. Rhomboid Major/Minor 14
      3. Supraspinatus 16
      4. Infraspinatus 16
      5. Serratus Anterior 18
      6. Pectoralis Major 20
      7. Latissimus Dorsi 22
      8. Intercostal Muscles (External) 24

III UPPER EXTREMITY 27

   A. Muscles
      1. Deltoid 28
      2. Coracobrachialis 30
      3. Biceps Brachii 32
      4. Brachialis 32
      5. Triceps Brachii 34
      6. Anconeus 35
      7. Brachioradialis 36
      8. Flexor Carpi Radialis 36
      9. Pronator Teres 37
     10. Flexor Carpi Ulnaris 38
     11. Flexor Digitorum Sublimis 39
     12. Flexor Digitorum Profundus 39
     13. Flexor Pollicis Longus 40
     14. Pronator Quadratus 41
     15. Extensor Carpi Radialis Longus and Brevis 42
     16. Extensor Digitorum Communis 42
     17. Extensor Carpi Ulnaris 42
     18. Supinator 46
     19. Extensor Pollicis Brevis 48
     20. Extensor Indicis Proprius 48
     21. Abductor Pollicis Longus 48
     22. Abductor Pollicis Brevis 50
     23. Flexor Pollicis Brevis 50
     24. Opponens Pollicis 50
     25. Abductor Digiti Quinti 52
     26. First Dorsal Interosseous 52
     27. Adductor Pollicis 52
     28. Lumbricales 54

B. Nerves 56
   1. Brachial Plexus—Diagram 58
   2. Brachial Plexus—Supraclavicular Fossa 58
               Erb's Point 60
   3. Brachial Plexus—Lower Plexus and Roots of the Peripheral 60
               Nerves in Axilla 62
   4. Median N—Diagram 64
   5. Ligament of Struthers 66
   6. Pronator Syndrome 68
   7. Anterior Interosseous Syndrome 70
   8. Ulnar N—Diagram 70
     a. Thoracic Outlet Compression 70
     b. Cubital Tunnel 70
     c. Guyon's Canal 72
   9. Radial N—Diagram 72
     a. Saturday Night Palsy 72
     b. Posterior Interosseous Syndrome 74
  10. Radial N—Level of Supinator 76
  11. Radial N—Forearm 78
  12. Radial N—Above Radial Styloid 80
  13. Cross Section: Level at Mid-arm 82
  14. Cross Section: Level at Epicondyle 84
  15. Cross Section: Level at Mid-forearm 86
  16. Cross Section: Level at Radial Styloid 88
  17. Cross Section: Level at Distal Carpal Bones (Carpal Tunnel) 90
  18. Cross Section: Level at Digit ....

IV TRUNK, PELVIC GIRDLE AND PERINEUM 93
  A. Muscles
    1. Paraspinal Lumbar Muscles 94
    2. Abdominal Muscles 96
      a. External Oblique 96
      b. Rectus Abdominus 96
    3. External Anal Sphincter 98

V LOWER EXTREMITY 101
  A. Muscles
    1. Iliopsoas 102
    2. Tensor Fasciae Latae 106
    3. Gluteus Maximus and Medius 108
    4. Biceps Femoris—Short Head 110
    5. Both Hamstrings 112
    6. Adductor Longus and Magnus 112
    7. Sartorius 112
    8. Quadriceps Femoris 112
    9. Anterior Tibial 114
   10. Extensor Digitorum Longus 114
   11. Peroneus Longus and Brevis 114
   12. Extensor Hallucis Longus 116
   13. Popliteus 117
   14. Gastrocnemius and Soleus 118
   15. Abductor Hallucis 120
   16. Abductor Digiti Quinti 120
   17. Flexor Digitorum Brevis 120
   18. Extensor Digitorum Brevis 122
   19. Tibialis Posterior 124

B. Nerves
1. Sacral Plexus—Diagram 126
2. Sciatic N
   a. At notch 128
   b. Electrostimulation 128
3. Lumbosacral Plexus—Diagram 130
4. Obturator N—Diagram 131
5. Lateral Femoral Cutaneous N—Diagram 131
6. Femoral N—Diagram 132
7. Saphenous N—Diagram 134
8. Sural N—Diagram 136
9. Posterior Tibial N—Diagram 138
10. Peroneal N—Diagram 140
11. Lateral and Medial Plantar N—Diagram 142
12. Cross Section: Level at Pubic Tubercle 144
13. Cross Section: Level at Mid-Thigh 146
14. Cross Section: Level at Upper Third of Patella 147
15. Cross Section: Level at Head of Fibula 148
16. Cross Section: Level at Mid-leg 149
17. Cross Section: Level Above Malleolus 150
18. Cross Section: Level at Forefoot 151

part I

HEAD and
NECK

I A 1 SUPERFICIAL MUSCLES OF FACE
I A 2 MASSETER

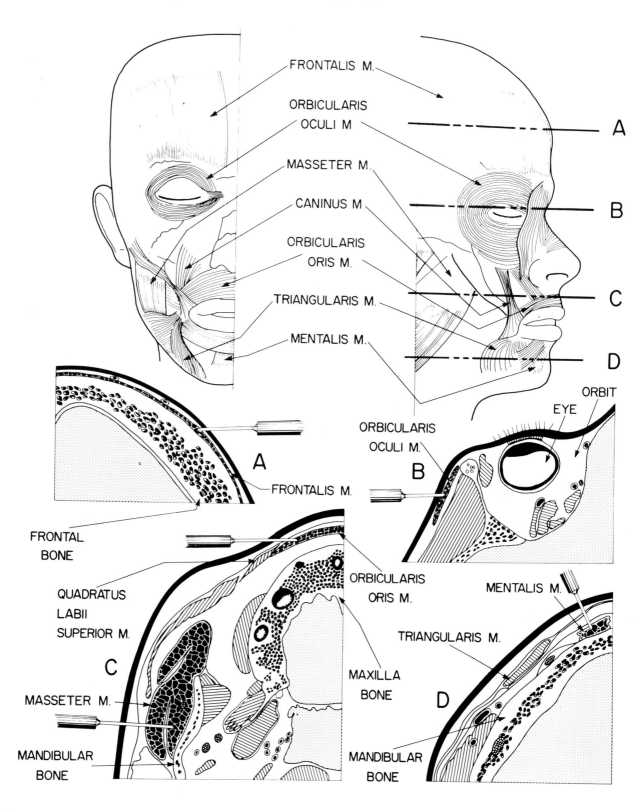

FRONTALIS M.

ORBICULARIS
OCULI M

MASSETER M.

CANINUS M

ORBICULARIS
ORIS M.

TRIANGULARIS M.

MENTALIS M.

A

B

C

D

ORBIT

EYE

ORBICULARIS
OCULI M.

B

A

FRONTALIS M.

FRONTAL
BONE

QUADRATUS
LABII
SUPERIOR M.

C

MASSETER M.

MANDIBULAR
BONE

ORBICULARIS
ORIS M.

MAXILLA
BONE

MENTALIS M.

TRIANGULARIS M.

D

MANDIBULAR
BONE

I A 1   Superficial muscles of the face
   a. Orbicularis oris
   b. Orbicularis oculi
   c. Frontalis
   d. Mentalis

Nerve Supply: Facial N (N VII)

Action: All are muscles of expression; specifically (a) closes and purses the lips, (b) closes the eye, (c) wrinkles and raises the brow, and (d) dimples the chin and raises the lower lip

The muscles innervated by the facial nerve are thin slips which must be carefully probed with the needle electrode; penetration through the mucous membrane is a common occurrence. The frontalis is located directly under the skin just above the frontal bone (a). The obicularis oculi is entered by carefully threading the electrode subcutaneously from the lateral region of the orbit (b). Study of the orbicularis oris is made somewhat simpler when the examiner holds the patient's lip between his own first and second fingers and slips the electrode into the intervening muscle tissue. Penetration is usually made at the angle of the mouth where the oris is joined by the caninus. The mentalis is a fairly isolated representative of innervation by the buccal branch of the facial nerve and is entered on either side of the midline of the chin (d).

In examining facial muscles, it is well to stay away from the midline since cross over may occur in the normal person as well as a sequel in reinnervation.

I A 2   Masseter

Nerve Supply: Anterior and posterior deep temporal nerves of the mandibular portion of the trigeminal nerve

Action: Closes the jaw

The masseter can be easily palpated when the teeth are forcibly clenched. The electrode is inserted on a line at right angles to the ramus of the mandible on a level with the anterior border of the pinna of the ear. During stimulation of the facial nerve, if the intensity of current is sufficiently high, a contraction of the masseter may ensue and mistakenly can be interpreted as a response of the facial muscles.

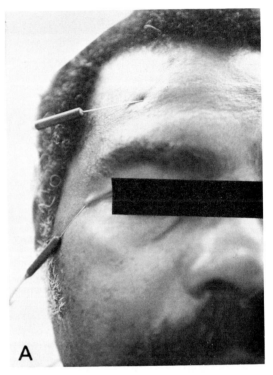

(A) Electrode inserted into frontalis M and obicularis oculi M.

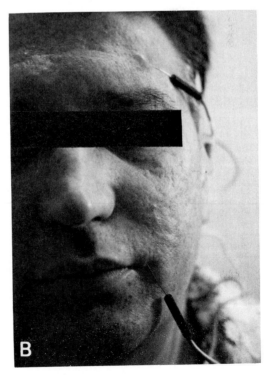

(B) Electrode inserted in the fronatlis M and the obicularis oris M.

I A 3   POSTERIOR AURICULAR

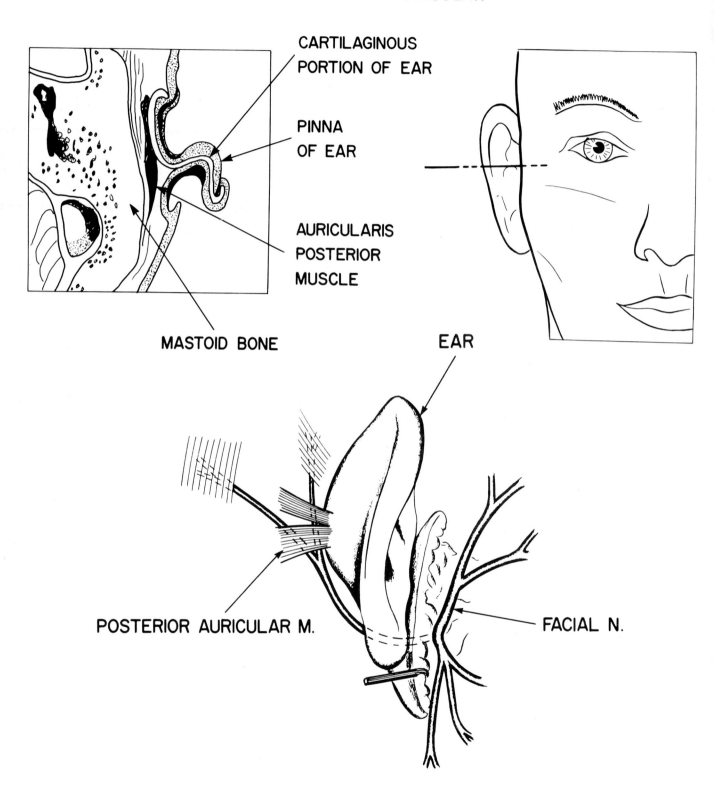

CARTILAGINOUS
PORTION OF EAR

PINNA
OF EAR

AURICULARIS
POSTERIOR
MUSCLE

MASTOID BONE

EAR

POSTERIOR AURICULAR M.

FACIAL N.

I A 3 Posterior auricular

Nerve Supply: Facial N (N VII), posterior auricular branch

Action: Draws ear backward, or, if there is any function at all, it is most commonly associated with movement of the scalp

It is well known that most people cannot voluntarily control this muscle. Nevertheless, it is useful to study the responses of the posterior auricular M in assessment of facial nerve electrostimulation since it is innervated by the first muscular branch of the facial N after its exit from the stylomastoid foramen. The muscle is located at the mid-position of the posterior aspect of the pinna. Needle electrode insertion is made into the fold which is accentuated by pulling the ear forward. The muscle is located within the skin redundancy.

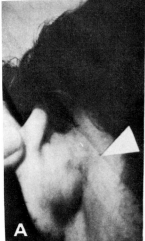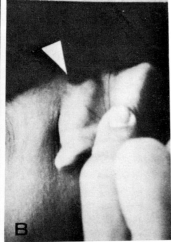

Surface view of the posterior aspect of the pinna. The *arrow* is pointing to the skin fold which contains the auricularis posterior M. In *A*, the muscle belly is prominent; the patient was an "ear wiggler."

I A 4 TONGUE

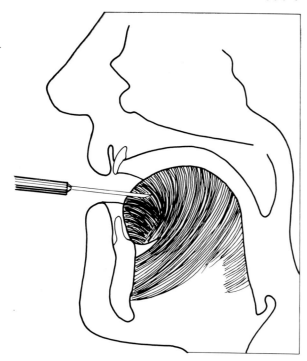 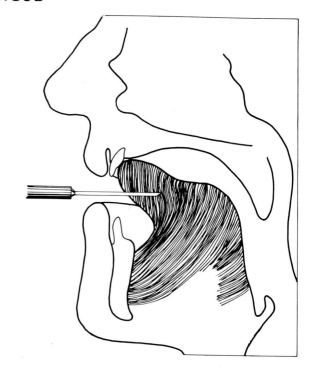

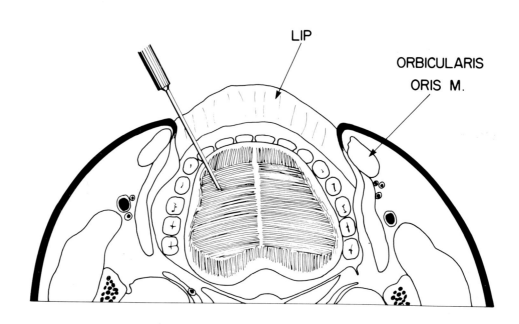

LIP

ORBICULARIS ORIS M.

I A 4   Tongue

Nerve Supply: Hypoglossal N (N XII)

Action: Because of the multiple number of muscles contributing to the architecture of the tongue, there are numerous and complicated movements which can be related mainly to the muscle fiber directions. For electromyographic (EMG) purposes, protrusion and side-to-side movement are most informative actions

The tongue should be examined in at least four sites: left and right halves of both the surface and underside. In most cases, a sharp electrode will easily and painlessly penetrate the surface of the tongue when it is resting in the floor of the mouth or will enter the underside of the muscle with the same ease when the mouth is opened and the tip of the tongue touched to the upper incisors. In some cases, it may be necessary to place a soft padding over the lower incisors and to gently hold the protruded tongue with a piece of gauze.

Examination of the tongue often is not as informative as one would like because so many persons are unable to completely relax this structure—especially with a needle electrode in place! The tendency to quivering, however, is minimized when the electrode is inserted into the undersurface—interpretation of the spontaneous activity is considerably enhanced when this approach is used.

I A 5 STERNOCLEIDOMASTOID
I A 6 LEVATOR SCAPULAE

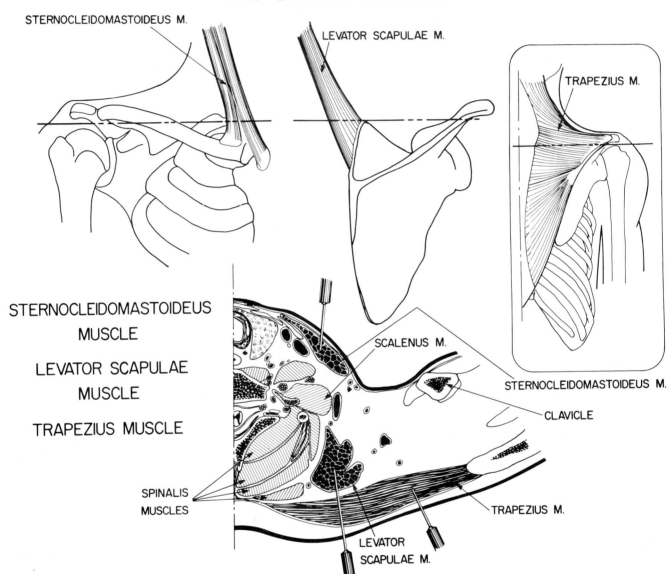

STERNOCLEIDOMASTOIDEUS M.

LEVATOR SCAPULAE M.

TRAPEZIUS M.

STERNOCLEIDOMASTOIDEUS
MUSCLE

LEVATOR SCAPULAE
MUSCLE

TRAPEZIUS MUSCLE

SCALENUS M.

STERNOCLEIDOMASTOIDEUS M.

CLAVICLE

SPINALIS
MUSCLES

LEVATOR
SCAPULAE M.

TRAPEZIUS M.

I A 5   Sternocleidomastoid

Nerve Supply: Accessory N (spinal portion) C_2, C_3

Action: One-sided action bends vertebral column and rotates head to opposite side; bilateral action bends head forward while lifting chin, forward flexes vertebral column

The thickest part of this most prominent neck muscle is at its middle portion so that electrode penetration is most reliable at this point. The muscle lies superficially.

I A 6   Levator scapulae

Nerve Supply: C_3, C_4 (C_5 through dorsal scapular N)

Action: Elevation of the superior angle of the scapula and fixes this angle as a fulcrum during upward rotation of the scapula

There is really little need to examine the levator scapulae since the C_3, C_4 spinal N distribution is examined more easily with other muscles (i.e., cervical paraspinal M). When the trapezius is atrophied, however, the levator becomes more prominent and is often mistaken for an intact portion of trapezius. It is identified by its angular direction between the upper cervical vertebrae and the superior angle of the scapula and its described action. In the illustration, as a matter of completion and orientation, a needle electrode is shown in the middle portion of the trapezius which is superficial to the levator scapulae.

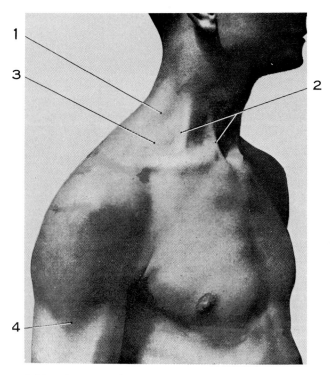

1, Edge of trapezius; *2*, sternocleidomastoid M, clavicular and sternal heads; *3*, supraclavicular fossa; and *4*, insertion of deltoid M. (From W. J. Hamilton, G. Simon, and S. G. Ian Hamilton: *Surface and Radiological Anatomy for Students and General Practitioners*, Ed. 5, Cambrdige, England: W. Heffer and Sons Ltd., 1971.)

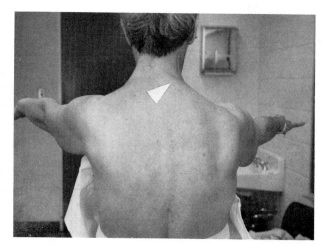

The upper trapezius M on the right is severely atrophied permitting easy visualization of the edge of the levator scapulae N.

I A 7 CERVICAL PARASPINAL

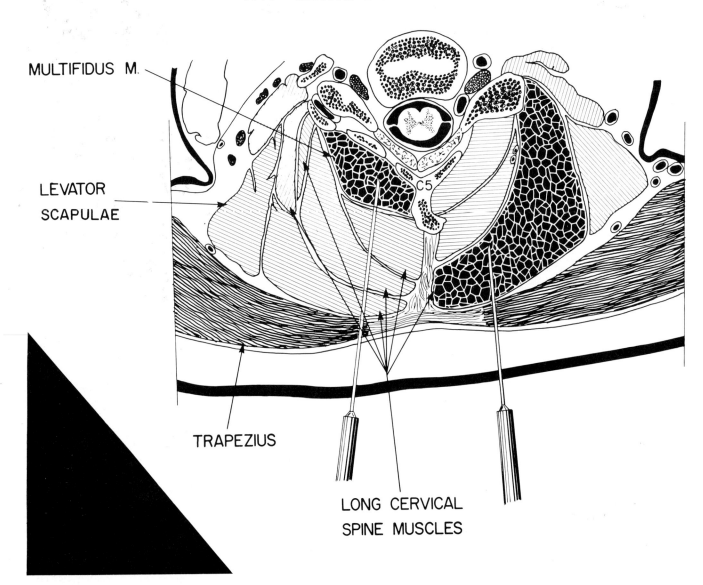

MULTIFIDUS M.

LEVATOR
SCAPULAE

C5

TRAPEZIUS

LONG CERVICAL
SPINE MUSCLES

I A 7   Cervical paraspinal muscles

Nerve Supply: Segmental nerves (posterior rami) of the region. The short muscles are fairly discretely supplied, but the long muscle innervation shows overlapping of at least 1 or 2 segments

Action: Extension and rotation of the spine and head (i.e., multifidus rotates the vertebra to the opposite side)

The short rotators and multifidus are deep and are probed by inserting the electrode just lateral to the spinous process and sliding the electrode down toward the lamina and transverse process. It is obvious that the multifidus cannot be clearly separated from the small rotators and segmental muscles (i.e., intertransversarii) but this matter is of little consequence since the interpretation is the same. The approach is entirely blind and is not infrequently painful, especially if a root is inadvertently touched. The long spinal muscles (splenius, longissimus, etc.) form rather prominent masses extending for several centimeters to either side of the spinous processes and ligamentum nuchae.

In order to attain complete relaxation of the patient, it is imperative to have the subject in a comfortable position—on his abdomen propped on pillows, or what appears to be best for the cervical area, a side-lying position with good support of head, neck and shoulders.

part II

PECTORAL GIRDLE and THORAX

II A 1 TRAPEZIUS
II A 2 RHOMBOID MAJOR/MINOR

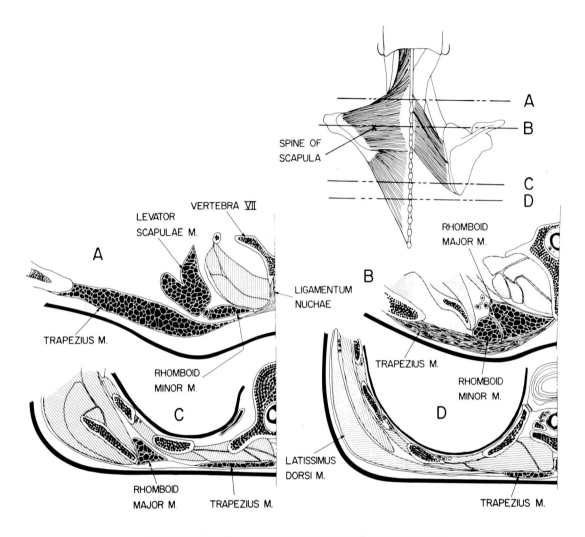

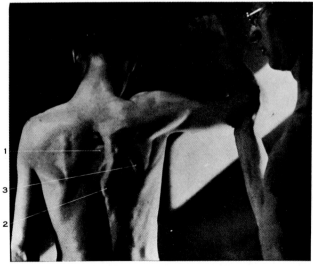

1, Middle trapezius; *2*, lower trapezius; and *3*, border of scapula. (From R. D. Lockhart: *Living Anatomy*, Ed. 5, London: Faber and Faber, Ltd., 1959.)

II A 1   Trapezius

Nerve Supply: Dual supply from spinal accessory N, and C_2, C_3, and C_4 (probably only muscle afferent fibers)

Action: Retracts the scapula, elevates lateral angle of scapula, and upward rotation of scapula

The broad trapezius muscle is best examined in its middle portion on a line with the spine of the scapula. Here it is superficial and practically covers the other back muscles. The lower fibers converge to the vertebral spines so that at level D there is so very little muscle bulk that erroneous needle insertion may occur frequently. This is especially true in the presence of atrophy when the muscle is extremely thinned out.

II A 2   Rhomboidii

Nerve Supply: Dorsal scapular N and C_5

Action: Retracts scapula, elevation of vertebral border of scapula

Except for a small portion of the rhomboid major which is just visible at the lower vertebral border of the scapula, the rhomboids are covered by the trapezius and cannot be penetrated in isolation with absolute assurance. When there is trapezius atrophy, the rhomboid muscles are prominent; the upward lateral to medial coursing of their fibers is identified by muscle testing. Since the innervation is usually only through C_5 (see "Brachial Plexus," p. 56), an isolated lesion of this single root may be identified by insertion of the electrode through the trapezius into the rhomboids in the hopes of demonstrating the presence of abnormal spontaneous activity. Negative findings are, of course, inconclusive. The portion of the rhomboid major which is not covered by the trapezius may be studied by insertion of the needle just lateral to the trapezius along the lower one-fourth of the vertebral border (C).

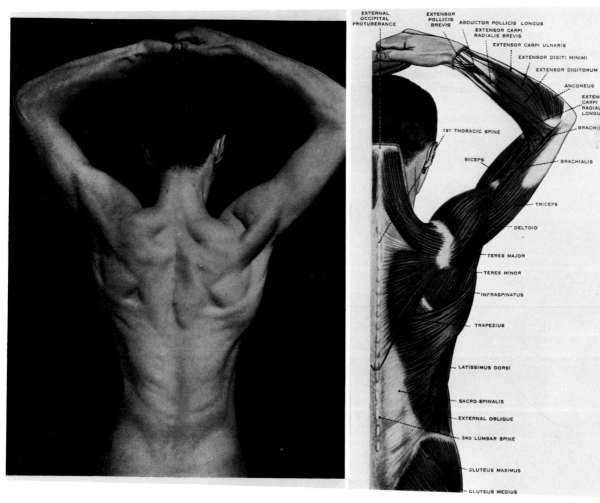

(From W. J. Hamilton, G. Simon, and S. G. Ian Hamilton: *Surface and Radiological Anatomy for Students and General Practitioners*, Ed. 5, Cambridge, England: W. Heffer and Sons Ltd., 1971.)

II A 3 SUPRASPINATUS
II A 4 INFRASPINATUS

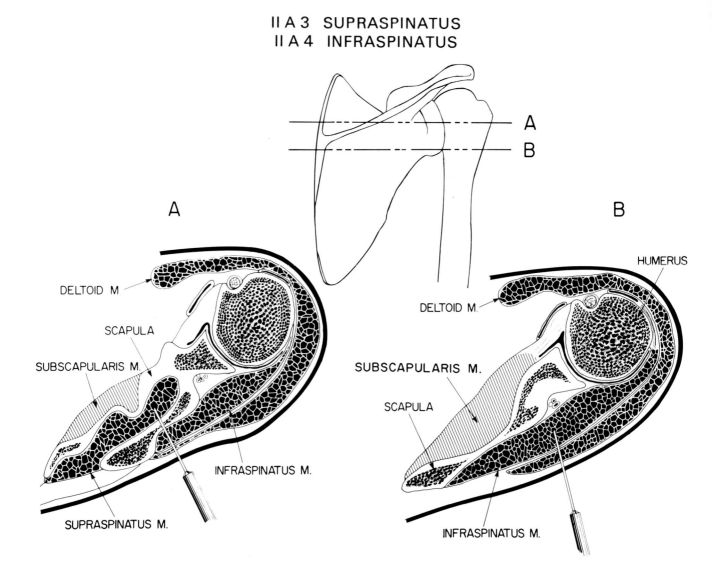

A

DELTOID M.

SCAPULA

SUBSCAPULARIS M.

INFRASPINATUS M.

SUPRASPINATUS M.

B

HUMERUS

DELTOID M.

SUBSCAPULARIS M.

SCAPULA

INFRASPINATUS M.

II A 3   Supraspinatus

Nerve Supply: Suprascapular N
C_5, C_6

Action: Abductor of arm

The needle electrode is introduced into the supraspinatus M after identification of the supraspinatus fossa by delineating the superior edge of the spine of the scapula. The needle is inserted perpendicularly at a central point in the fossa until it strikes the bone and then is slightly withdrawn to lie in the muscle.

II A 4   Infraspinatus

Nerve Supply: Suprascapular N
C_5, C_6

Action: External rotation of humerus

The region of the infraspinous fossa which is below the bony landmark is also identified by palpation of the spine of the scapula. The needle electrode is inserted perpendicularly down to the plate of the bone and slightly withdrawn to lie in the muscle.

II A 5 SERRATUS ANTERIOR

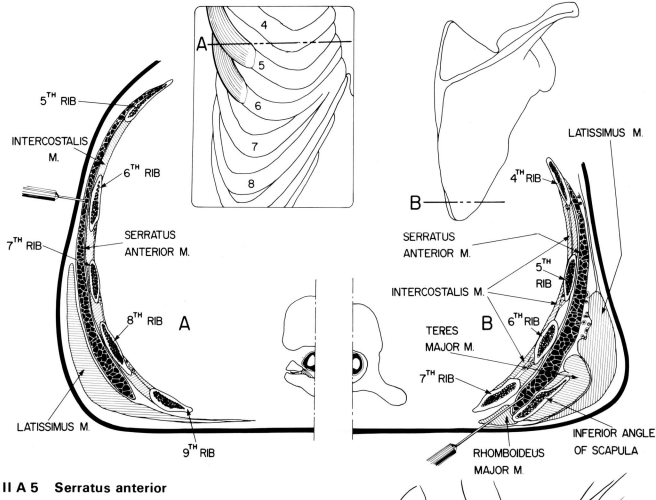

II A 5   Serratus anterior

Nerve Supply: Long thoracic N
C_5, C_6, and C_7

Action: Protraction of the shoulder, especially inferior angle; holds the scapula tightly against ribs

The serratus anterior may be examined in two ways. (1) The muscle may be entered in the mid-axillary line on a level with the 6th rib. Penetration is made exactly opposite the rib which is identified by placing fingers above and below in the 5th and 6th intercostal spaces, respectively. The maneuver obviates inapparent penetration of the thorax (pneumothorax!). (2) The muscle may also be examined at the vertebral border of the inferior angle of the scapula. This edge is rotated laterally by sliding the internally rotated arm across the back toward the midline. Since the long thoracic nerve is derived directly from the anterior rami of C_5, C_6, and C_7, examination of the serratus anterior affords an opportunity to identify highest level plexus lesions (e.g., traction avulsion).

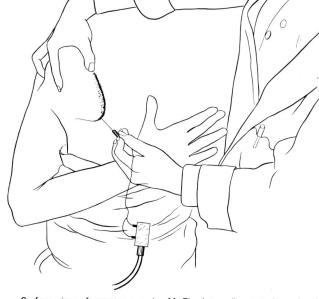

Surface view of serratus anterior M. The internally rotated arm is slid across the back toward the midline, bringing the inferior angle of the scapula into a "winged" position. The needle electrode is slipped in anteriorly to the edge of the angle of the bone.

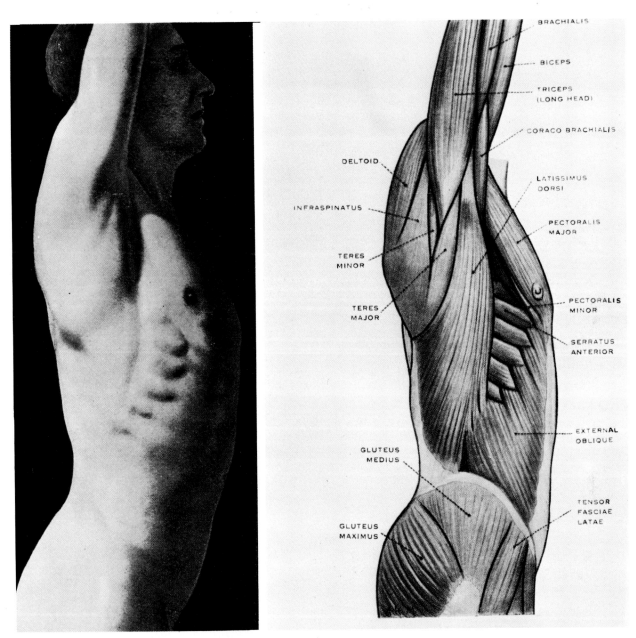

(From W. J. Hamilton, G. Simon, and S. G. Ian Hamilton: *Surface and Radiological Anatomy for Students and General Practitioners*, Ed. 5, Cambridge, England: W. Heffer and Sons Ltd., 1971.)

II A 6 PECTORALIS MAJOR

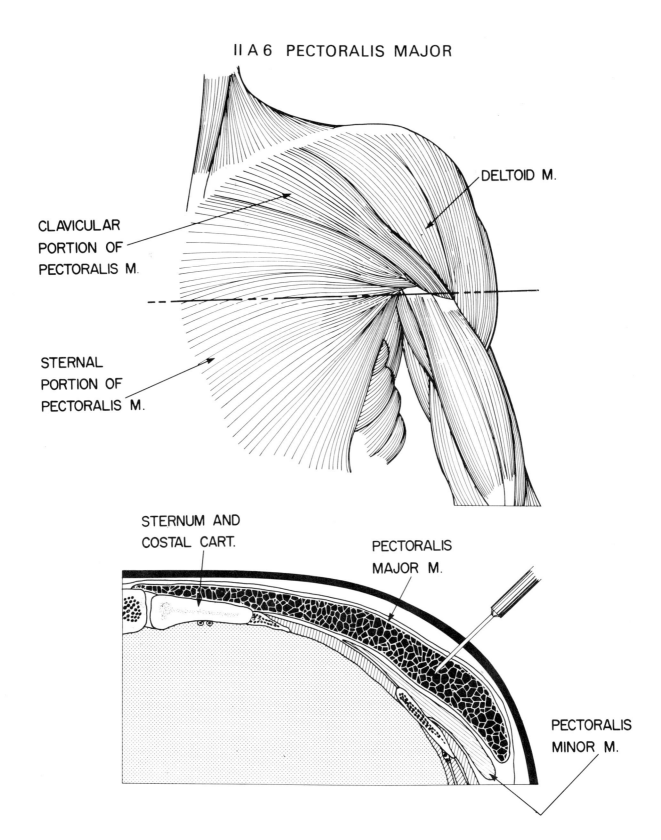

DELTOID M.

CLAVICULAR PORTION OF PECTORALIS M.

STERNAL PORTION OF PECTORALIS M.

STERNUM AND COSTAL CART.

PECTORALIS MAJOR M.

PECTORALIS MINOR M.

II A 6   Pectoralis major

Nerve Supply: Dual supply from medial (C_8 to T_1) and lateral (C_5 to C_7) anterior thoracic N

Action: Adduction of the arm

The pectoralis major practically covers the front of the chest extending laterally to form the anterior axillary line. The muscle belly is identified by pinching the anterior axillary fold between the fingers of the examiner and inserting the electrode into the belly of the muscle about 2 or 3 cm medially and 2 or 3 cm above the nipple line. The approach into the muscle is from lateral to medial, avoiding the level of the rib cage.

II A 7 LATISSIMUS DORSI
LEVEL: JUST BELOW XIPHISTERNAL JOINT—T10

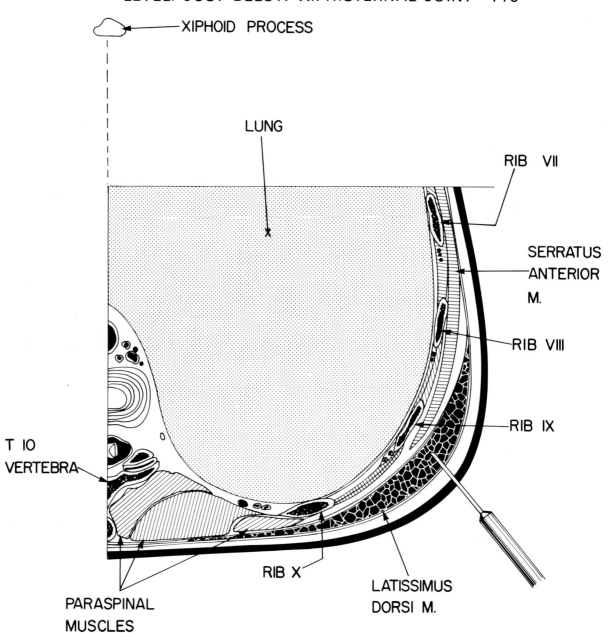

XIPHOID PROCESS

LUNG

RIB VII

SERRATUS ANTERIOR M.

RIB VIII

RIB IX

T 10 VERTEBRA

RIB X

LATISSIMUS DORSI M.

PARASPINAL MUSCLES

II A 7   Latissimus dorsi

Nerve Supply: Thoracodorsal N
(C$_6$), C$_7$, and (C$_8$)

Action: Adduction
Inward rotation of arm
Extension of arm

The latissimus dorsi complements the trapezius in its broad coverage of the back. At the level of a line between the xiphoid-manubrial junction anteriorly and the spine of D$_{10}$, the latissimus is not covered by another muscle. The electrode can be inserted into the muscle in this region; frequently the muscle edge can be seen and palpated since the margin runs up to form the outer edge of the posterior wall of the axilla. From the viewpoint of clinical electromyography, examination of the latissimus or the pectoralis is not called for frequently unless the concern is investigation of fairly isolated lesions.

II A 8 INTERCOSTAL

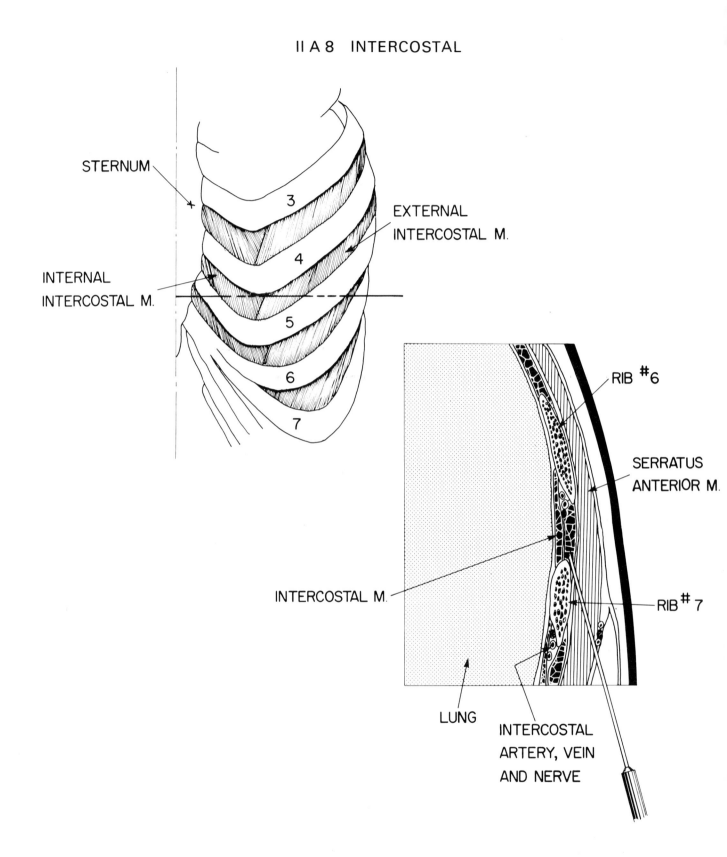

STERNUM

EXTERNAL INTERCOSTAL M.

INTERNAL INTERCOSTAL M.

3

4

5

6

7

RIB #6

SERRATUS ANTERIOR M.

INTERCOSTAL M.

RIB #7

LUNG

INTERCOSTAL ARTERY, VEIN AND NERVE

II A 8   External intercostal muscles

Nerve Supply: Regional intercostal N

Action: Elevation of the ribs

The electrode is inserted into the external intercostal M in the region of the mid-axillary line. The needle is kept in the vertical plane of the ribs, hugging the anterosuperior margin of the bone. This maneuver will avoid the intercostal neurovascular bundle and as well avoid penetration of the pleural space. Even in the best of hands, the maneuver is delicate and faces the possibility of an inadvertent pneumothorax.

part III

UPPER EXTREMITY

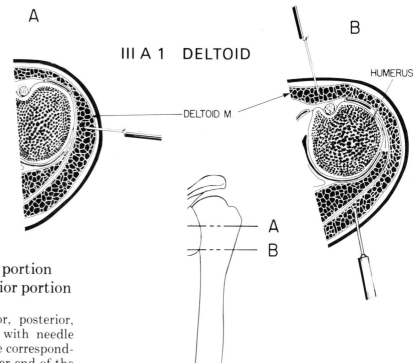

III A 1 DELTOID

III A 1   Deltoid

Nerve Supply: Axillary N
C_5, C_6

Action: Abduction
Flexion of arm—anterior portion
Extension of arm—posterior portion

Each portion of the deltoid—anterior, posterior, and middle bellies—can be examined with needle electrodes inserted perpendicularly to the corresponding surfaces of the humerus. At the upper end of the arm, there are no other muscles which interposes between the bone and the deltoid. The major depressions that divide the muscle into its identifiable portions can usually be palpated.

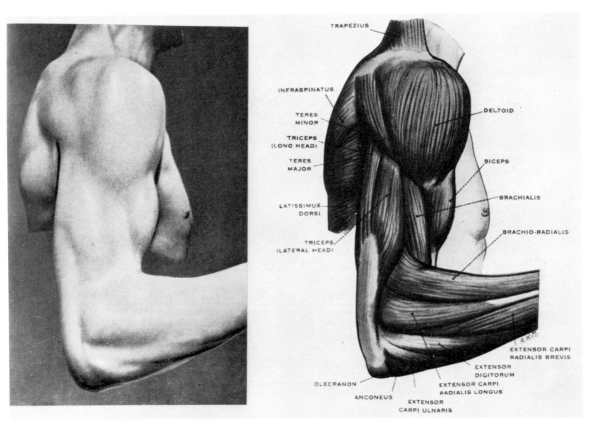

(From W. J. Hamilton, G. Simon, and S. G. Ian Hamilton: *Surface and Radiological Anatomy for Students and General Practitioners*, Ed. 5, Cambridge, England: W. Heffer and Sons Ltd., 1971.)

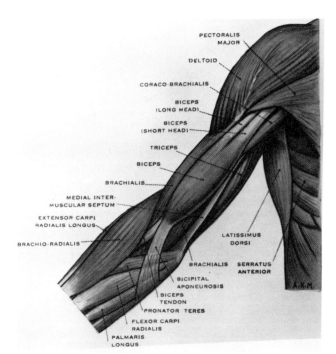

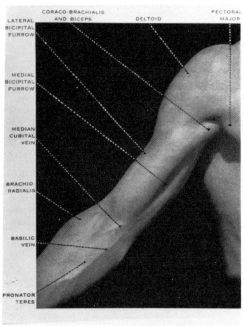

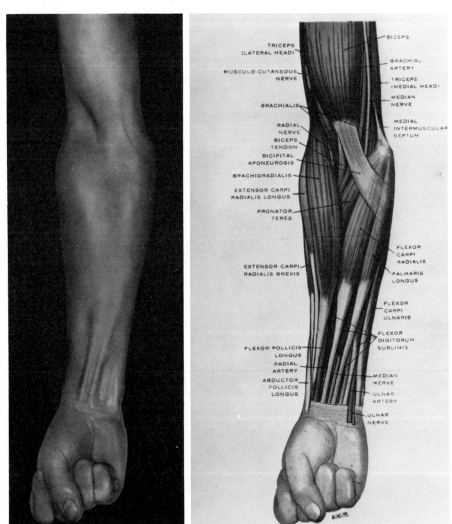

(From W. J. Hamilton, G. Simon, and S. G. Ian Hamilton: *Surface and Radiological Anatomy for Students and General Practitioners*, Ed. 5, Cambridge, England: W. Heffer and Sons Ltd., 1971).

29

III A 2 CORACORBRACHIALIS

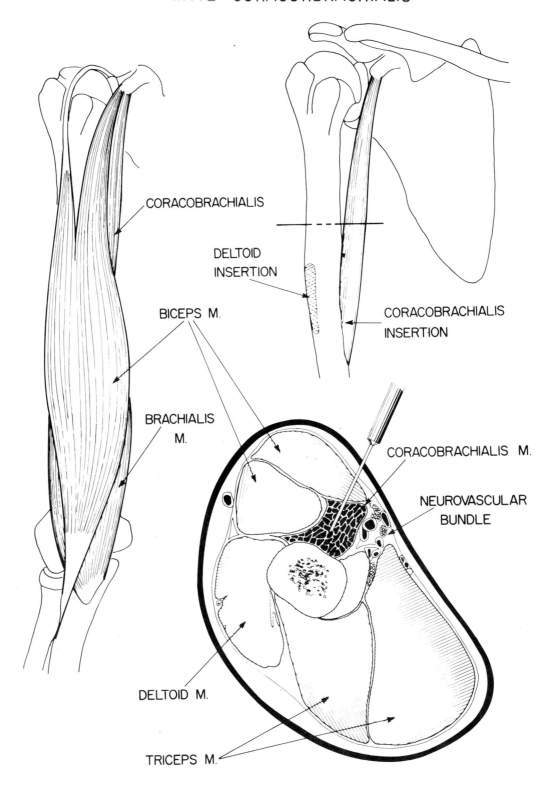

CORACOBRACHIALIS

DELTOID
INSERTION

CORACOBRACHIALIS
INSERTION

BICEPS M.

BRACHIALIS
M.

CORACOBRACHIALIS M.

NEUROVASCULAR
BUNDLE

DELTOID M.

TRICEPS M.

III A 2   Coracorbrachialis

Nerve Supply: Musculocutaneous N
C_6, C_7

Action: Flexion of the arm
Adduction of the arm

The bulge making up the coracobrachialis and the short head of the biceps brachii usually can be seen when the arm is abducted above the horizontal and externally rotated. The combined muscle mass can be palpated just posterior to the lateral margin of the pectoralis major and superior to the brachial neurovascular bundle.

This muscle is not examined frequently because sufficient information concerning the musculocutaneous nerve and C_6, C_7 may be readily obtained from more accessible structures. If the problem should concern precise localization of a lesion affecting the musculocutaneous nerve itself or the lateral cord of the brachial plexus, then examination of the coracobrachialis would be useful.

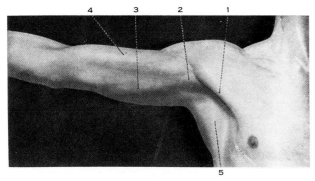

1, Pectoralis major; *2*, coracobrachialis, short head of the biceps; *3*, medial head of the triceps; *4*, biceps brachii, and *5*, latissimus dorsi. (Modified from W. J. Hamilton, G. Simon, and S. G. Ian Hamilton: *Surface and Radiological Anatomy for Students and General Practitioners*, Ed. 5, Cambridge, England: W. Heffer and Sons Ltd., 1971.)

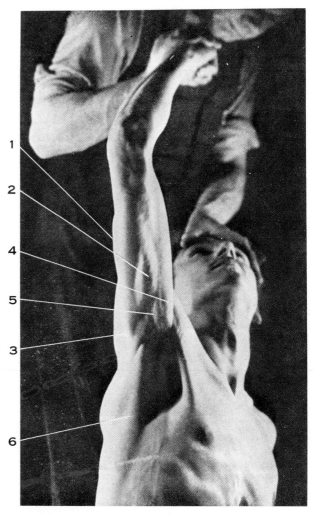

1, Triceps, lateral head; *2*, triceps, medial head; *3*, triceps, long head; *4*, coracobrachialis, short head of biceps; *5*, brachial neurovascular bundle, and *6*, latissimus dorsi. (From R. D. Lockhart: *Living Anatomy*, Ed. 5, London: Faber and Faber, Ltd., 1959.)

III A 3 BICEPS BRACHII
III A 4 BRACHIALIS

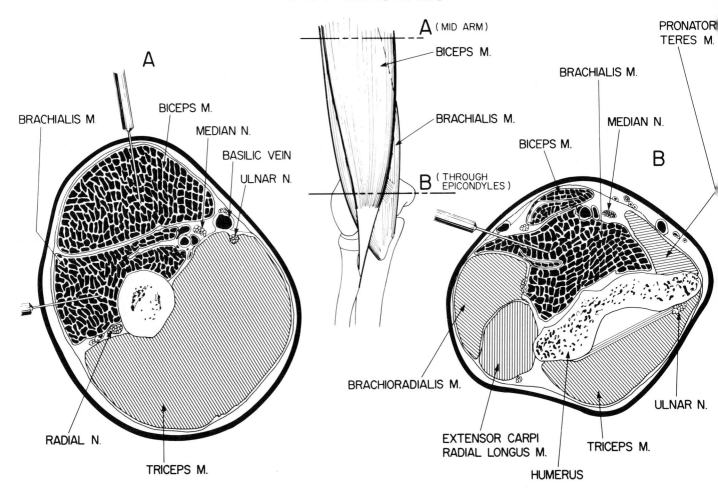

A

BRACHIALIS M.

BICEPS M.

MEDIAN N.

BASILIC VEIN

ULNAR N.

RADIAL N.

TRICEPS M.

A (MID ARM)

BICEPS M.

BRACHIALIS M.

B (THROUGH EPICONDYLES)

PRONATOR TERES M.

BRACHIALIS M.

MEDIAN N.

BICEPS M.

B

BRACHIORADIALIS M.

EXTENSOR CARPI RADIAL LONGUS M.

HUMERUS

TRICEPS M.

ULNAR N.

III A 3   Biceps brachii

Nerve Supply: Musculocutaneous N
C_5, C_6

Action: Flexion of the forearm on arm
Supination of forearm

The biceps brachii is the most prominent muscle of the anterior surface of the brachium. The middle of the belly (A) formed by the two heads is most conveniently examined although one must bear in mind that the coincidence of the zone of innervation in this region enhances the possibility of encountering end plate potential activity.

III A 4   Brachialis

Nerve Supply: Musculocutaneous N
C_5, C_6
Radial N (to the lower lateral portion of the muscle)

Action: Flexion of elbow

The brachialis lies directly on the humerus and is entered best with the electrode at level B. At this point, the biceps has become almost tendinous and is of relatively small girth. The needle is directed down and medially into the brachialis from the lateral margin of the biceps.

III A 5   TRICEPS

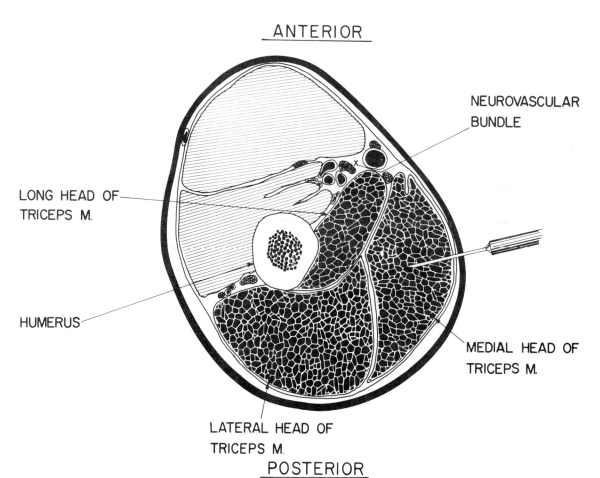

ANTERIOR

NEUROVASCULAR
BUNDLE

LONG HEAD OF
TRICEPS M.

HUMERUS

MEDIAL HEAD OF
TRICEPS M.

LATERAL HEAD OF
TRICEPS M.

POSTERIOR

III A 5   Triceps

Nerve Supply: Radial N
C_6, C_7, and C_8

Action: Extensor of the forearm

The three heads of the triceps are rather distinct and can be examined in fairly isolated fashion. Needle insertion is carried out with reference as shown in the topographical figure on p. 31. A major branch of the radial nerve to the long head forms in the axilla so that only partial denervation of this portion of the muscle may occur even with a high lesion of the radial nerve in the arm. Except for such problems of exact localization of a radial nerve lesion and the desirability of thorough sampling, examination of distal and proximal parts of the muscle is quite sufficient. The cross section shown is located approximately 12 cm above the medial epicondyle (adult) at about mid arm.

III A 6 ANCONEUS

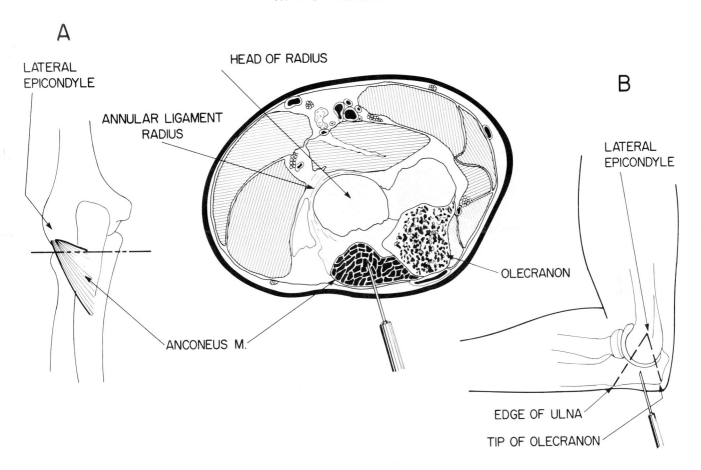

A

LATERAL EPICONDYLE

HEAD OF RADIUS

ANNULAR LIGAMENT RADIUS

ANCONEUS M.

B

LATERAL EPICONDYLE

OLECRANON

EDGE OF ULNA

TIP OF OLECRANON

III A 6 Anconeus

Nerve Supply: Radial N
C_6, C_7, and C_8

Action: Extension of the elbow

The anconeus muscle is small but its prominent subcutaneous position facilitates needle electrode examination. The lateral epicondyle and olecranon process of the ulna are palpated and the electrode is inserted into the roughly triangular space as outlined in *B*. The muscle is a good representative of the radial distribution and is innervated via a terminal of a branch to the medial belly of the triceps which originates above the level of the elbow joint.

III A 7 BRACHIORADIALIS
III A 8 FLEXOR CARPI RADIALIS

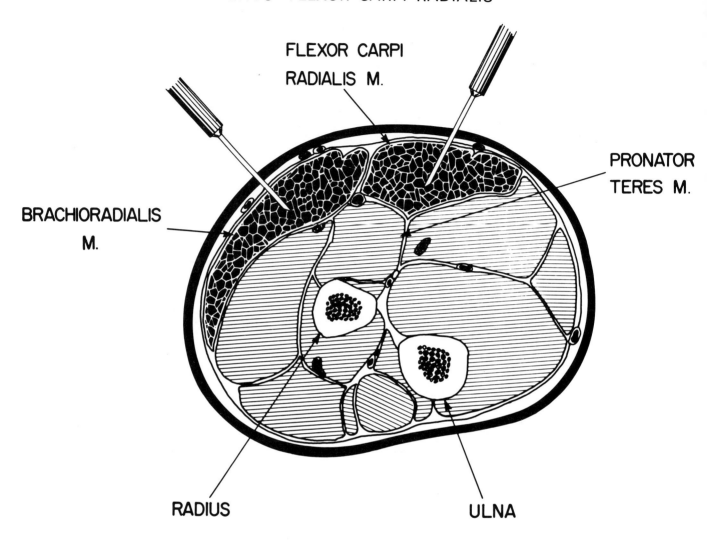

FLEXOR CARPI
RADIALIS M.

BRACHIORADIALIS
M.

PRONATOR
TERES M.

RADIUS

ULNA

III A 7   Brachioradialis

Nerve Supply: Radial N (above elbow)
C_5, C_6

Action: Flexion of the elbow

III A 8   Flexor carpi radialis

Nerve Supply: Median N
C_6, C_7

Action: Wrist flexion

The flexor carpi radialis is located in the middle third of the anterior forearm while the brachioradialis is really anterolateral in location and can easily be grasped between the examiner's thumb and index finger. The needle electrodes are introduced in the direction which the drawing indicates, keeping in mind the relatively superficial position of both muscles. At the *mid forearm* level at which the cross section is shown, the pronator teres is no longer superficial.

III A 9   PRONATOR TERES

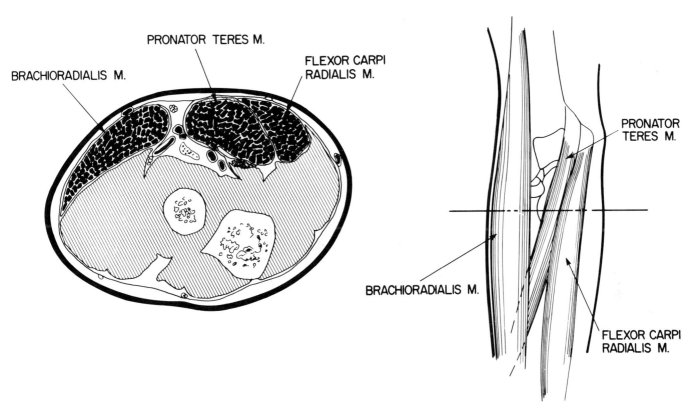

BRACHIORADIALIS M.

PRONATOR TERES M.

FLEXOR CARPI RADIALIS M.

PRONATOR TERES M.

BRACHIORADIALIS M.

FLEXOR CARPI RADIALIS M.

III A 9   Pronator teres

Nerve Supply: Median N (just distal to the entrance of the nerve between the ulnar and humeral heads of the muscle)
C_6, C_7

Action: Pronation of the forearm

At the level indicated (approximately 5 cm below the medial epicondyle) the brachioradialis and flexor carpi radialis muscles are prominent medially and laterally. The pronator runs just lateral to the flexor carpi radialis across the front of the forearm to about mid-forearm level. The needle electrode is inserted into the muscle belly about 1 cm lateral to the edge of the flexor carpi radialis. The lateral side of the pronator itself may be defined by palpation of the deep subcutaneous depression between the muscle and the brachioradialis.

III A 10 FLEXOR CARPI ULNARIS

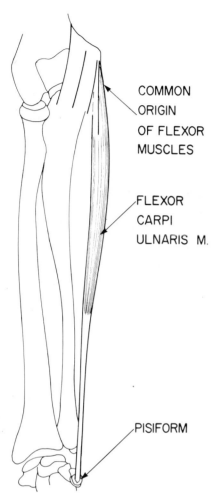

COMMON
ORIGIN
OF FLEXOR
MUSCLES

FLEXOR
CARPI
ULNARIS M.

PISIFORM

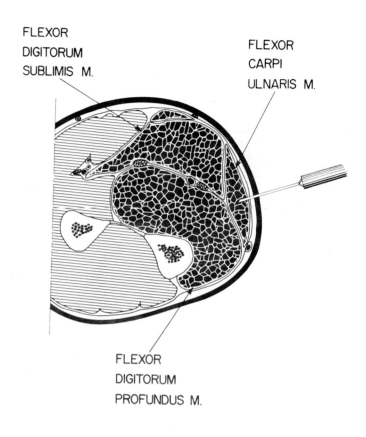

FLEXOR
DIGITORUM
SUBLIMIS M.

FLEXOR
CARPI
ULNARIS M.

FLEXOR
DIGITORUM
PROFUNDUS M.

**III A 10   Flexor carpi ulnaris
Mid-arm level**

Nerve Supply: Ulnar N
(C_7), C_8 to T_1

Action: Flexion of the wrist
Ulnar deviation of the wrist

The flexor carpi ulnaris is examined with the electrode inserted in a quite superficial position. (If electrical stimulation of the muscle is carried out, it can be observed that very frequently the needle goes completely through the muscle into the flexor digitorum profundus. Therefore, penetration should be kept relatively superficial and about a finger's breath

anterior to the anterior surface of the ulna.) The wedge-shaped muscle can be discretely palpated when the subject's fingers are relaxed and the wrist brought into sharp ulnar deviation. The innervation of the muscle usually arises just after the ulnar nerve passes between the two originating heads of the muscle but it may arise, as well, above the epicondyle so that involvement of the flexor carpi ulnaris is not a completely reliable differential index of above elbow vs. below elbow ulnar nerve lesions.

III A 11 FLEXOR DIGITORUM SUBLIMIS
III A 12 FLEXOR DIGITORUM PROFUNDUS

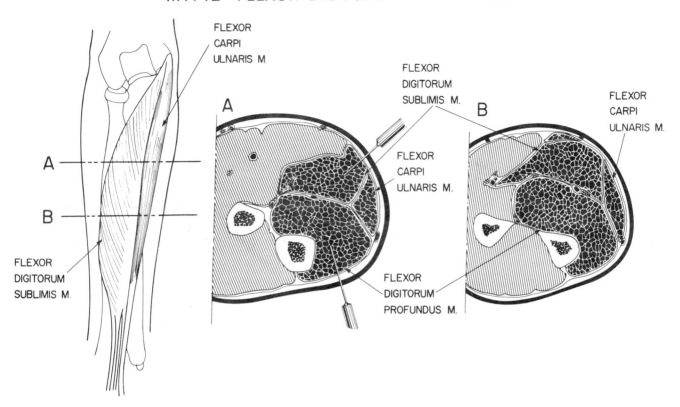

III A 11 Flexor digitorum sublimis

Nerve Supply: Median N
(C₇), C₈ to T₁

Action: Flexion of proximal interphalangeal joints

III A 12 Flexor digitorum profundus

Nerve Supply: (Double innervation—median supply is usually through the anterior interosseous N)
Median N
Ulnar N
(C₇), C₈ to T₁

With due regard to the wedge-shaped flexor carpi ulnaris which is interposed with its base facing medially, the superficial digital flexor muscle practically covers the profundus. When the flexor carpi ulnaris is identified by acute ulnar deviation of the wrist, the superficial flexor can be accurately penetrated by downward insertion of the electrode lateral to the upper margin of the flexor carpi ulnaris.

The profundus is entered by insertion of the electrode through the flexor carpi ulnaris down to the ulna and then slightly withdrawing the tip of the electrode back into the substance of the muscle or, as shown in A, the electrode can be inserted from a posteromedial direction toward the ulna.

III A 13   FLEXOR POLLICIS LONGUS

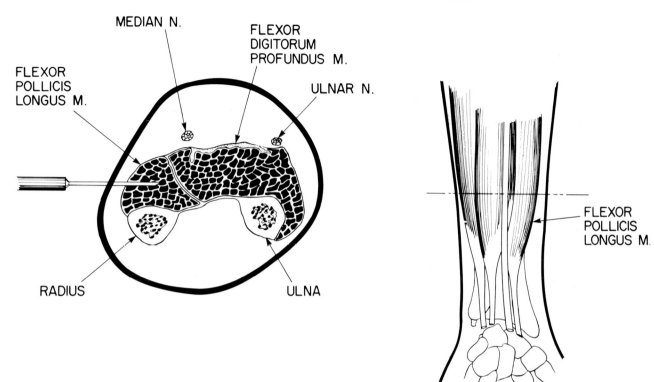

FLEXOR
POLLICIS
LONGUS M.

MEDIAN N.

FLEXOR
DIGITORUM
PROFUNDUS M.

ULNAR N.

RADIUS

ULNA

FLEXOR
POLLICIS
LONGUS M.

III A 13   Flexor pollicis longus

Nerve Supply: Median N (anterior interosseous branch)
(C_7), C_8 to T_1

Action: Flexion of distal joint of the thumb

The level indicated in the frontal section is about 10 to 12 cm above the radial styloid. Here the flexor pollicis longus covers the anterior surface of the radius. It may be entered with the electrode from the side as shown or vertically from above to lie just superior to the bone. This is an important muscle to examine in identification of the anterior interosseous nerve syndrome.

III A 14 PRONATOR QUADRATUS

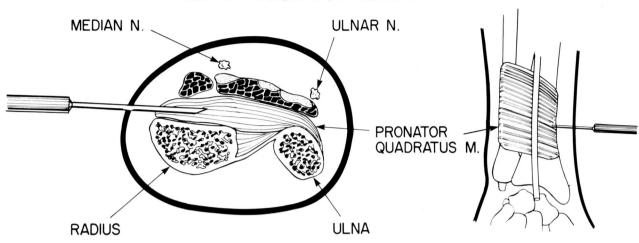

III A 14   Pronator quadratus

Nerve Supply: Median N (anterior interosseous branch)
(C$_7$), C$_8$ to T$_1$

Action: Pronation of the wrist

In examination of this flat muscle, which runs from the distal quarter of the ulna to the distal quarter of the radius, the electrode insertion must avoid the ulnar nerve and vessels, the radial artery and vein and the median nerve. This is accomplished by palpation of the radial and ulnar pulses and identification of the tendon of the flexor carpi ulnaris, flexor carpi radialis and palmaris longus at the wrist. From the radial side, the electrode is introduced in a horizontal plane about 5 cm above the styloid tip. The electrode is kept close to the anterior surface of the bone, but posterior to the vessels, and penetrates to a point somewhat lateral to the edge of the tendon of the palmaris longus.

III A 15 EXTENSOR CARPI RADIALIS BREVIS AND LONGUS
III A 16 EXTENSOR DIGITORUM COMMUNIS
III A 17 EXTENSOR CARPI ULNARIS

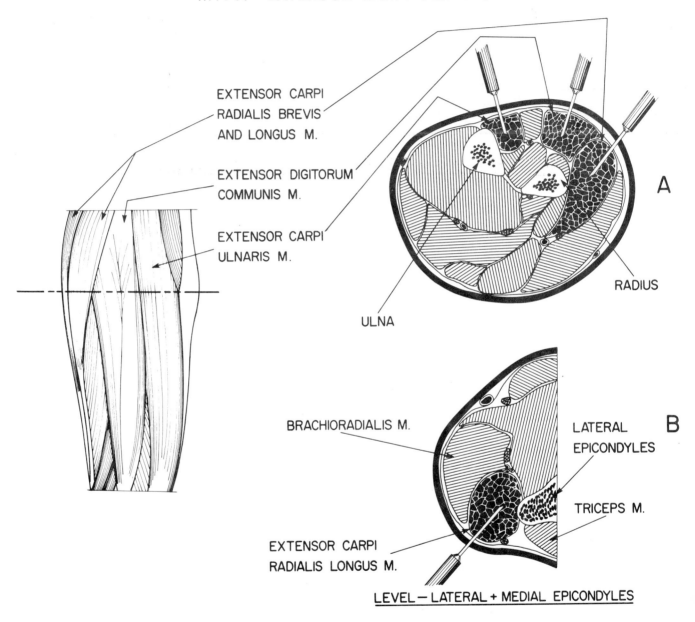

EXTENSOR CARPI
RADIALIS BREVIS
AND LONGUS M.

EXTENSOR DIGITORUM
COMMUNIS M.

EXTENSOR CARPI
ULNARIS M.

RADIUS

ULNA

A

BRACHIORADIALIS M.

LATERAL
EPICONDYLES

TRICEPS M.

EXTENSOR CARPI
RADIALIS LONGUS M.

B

LEVEL — LATERAL + MEDIAL EPICONDYLES

III A 15   Extensor carpi radialis longus

Nerve Supply: Radial N (branch above the lateral epicondyle) C_6, C_7

Action: Extension and radial abduction of wrist

Note: Becomes broad tendon in mid-arm level as does the brachioradialis.

III A 15   (a) Extensor carpi radialis brevis

Nerve Supply: Radial N (either the superficial or deep branch or the trunk just before bifurcation) C_6, C_7

Action: Extension of wrist

III A 16   Extensor digitorum communis

Nerve Supply: Radial N (deep branch after the nerve emerges from the supinator) C_6, C_7, and C_8

Action: Extension and abduction of the digits

III A 17   Extensor carpi ulnaris

Nerve Supply: Radial N (deep branch) (C_6), C_7, and C_8

Action: Extension of the wrist
  Ulnar deviation of the wrist

These superficial extensor muscles are shown in cross section at a level approximately 12 or 13 cm below the epicondyles. The extensor digitorum communis occupies the prominent central position, the ulnaris is most medially located and the radial extensors lie on a line with the brachioradialis and emerge along the posterior border of that muscle. Examination of the extensor digitorum which is most easily and accurately identified provides good representation of the condition of the C_6, C_7 root or the deep radial nerve distribution. However, where entrapment of the radial nerve as it penetrates the supinator muscle is suspected, then electromyographic (EMG) examination of the extensor carpi radialis longus which is innervated proximally and the extensor digitorum communis which is innervated distal to the supinator, may provide good differentiating information.

In cross section B through the epicondyle, the high origin of the extensor carpi radialis longus is shown; there is no confusion at this level with the extensor digitorum communis because the latter originates distally. When the belly of the brachioradialis is grasped between the examiner's fingers, then the extensor carpi radialis longus lies just medially and next to the lateral epicondyle.

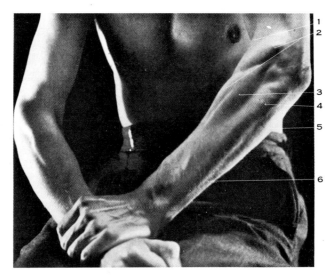

1, Brachioradialis; *2*, extensor carpi radialis longus and brevis; *3*, extensor digitorum communis; *4*, extensor carpi ulnaris; *5*, edge of flexor carpi ulnaris; and *6*, edge of ulna. (From R. D. Lockhart: *Living Anatomy*, Ed. 5, London: Faber and Faber, Ltd., 1959.)

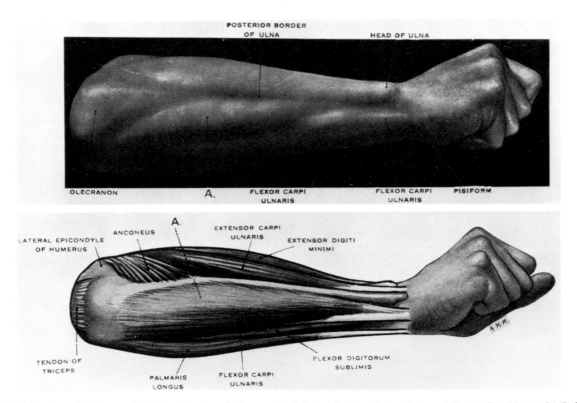

(From W. J. Hamilton, G. Simon, and S. G. Ian Hamilton: *Surface and Radiological Anatomy for Students and General Practitioners*, Ed. 5, Cambridge, England: W. Heffer and Sons Ltd., 1971.)

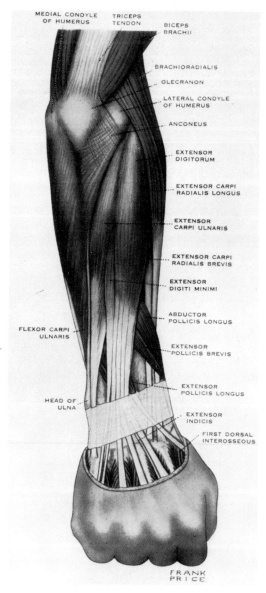

MEDIAL CONDYLE
OF HUMERUS

TRICEPS
TENDON

BICEPS
BRACHII

BRACHIORADIALIS

OLECRANON

LATERAL CONDYLE
OF HUMERUS

ANCONEUS

EXTENSOR
DIGITORUM

EXTENSOR CARPI
RADIALIS LONGUS

EXTENSOR
CARPI ULNARIS

EXTENSOR CARPI
RADIALIS BREVIS

EXTENSOR
DIGITI MINIMI

ABDUCTOR
POLLICIS LONGUS

FLEXOR CARPI
ULNARIS

EXTENSOR
POLLICIS BREVIS

EXTENSOR
POLLICIS LONGUS

HEAD OF
ULNA

EXTENSOR
INDICIS

FIRST DORSAL
INTEROSSEOUS

FRANK
PRICE.

(From W. J. Hamilton, G. Simon, and S. G. Ian Hamilton: *Surface and Radiological Anatomy for Students and General Practitioners*, Ed. 5, Cambridge, England: W. Heffer and Sons Ltd., 1971.)

III A 18 SUPINATOR

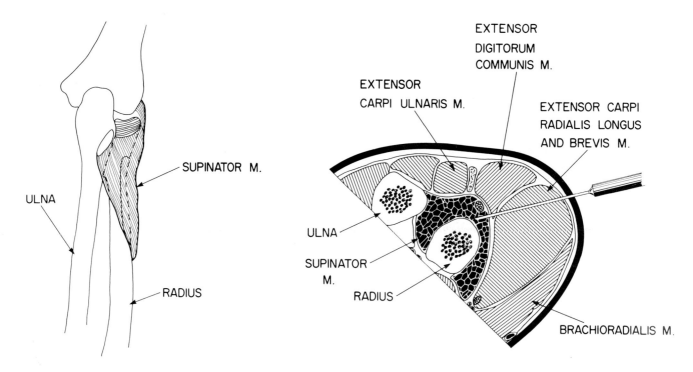

SUPINATOR M.

ULNA

RADIUS

EXTENSOR
DIGITORUM
COMMUNIS M.

EXTENSOR
CARPI ULNARIS M.

EXTENSOR CARPI
RADIALIS LONGUS
AND BREVIS M.

ULNA

SUPINATOR
M.

RADIUS

BRACHIORADIALIS M.

III A 18   Supinator

Nerve Supply: Radial N (deep branch—at a point just above the muscle or as the nerve passes through the muscle)
C_6, C_7

Action: Supinator of the forearm

Examination of the supinator muscle provides no more additional information regarding the C_6, C_7 rami or the radial nerve than examination of some of the other muscles of this innervation other than some precise data requested in specific cases (e.g., level of injury to the radial nerve). Although the muscle is a deep one, the EMG examination is not difficult since the muscle envelops the radius. It is entered with the electrode at a level just below the neck of the radius (about 6 or 7 cm below the epicondyle). The needle is inserted down to the bone and slightly withdrawn into the substance of the muscle.

III A 19   EXTENSOR POLLICIS BREVIS
III A 20   EXTENSOR INDICIS PROPRIUS
III A 21   ABDUCTOR POLLICIS LONGUS

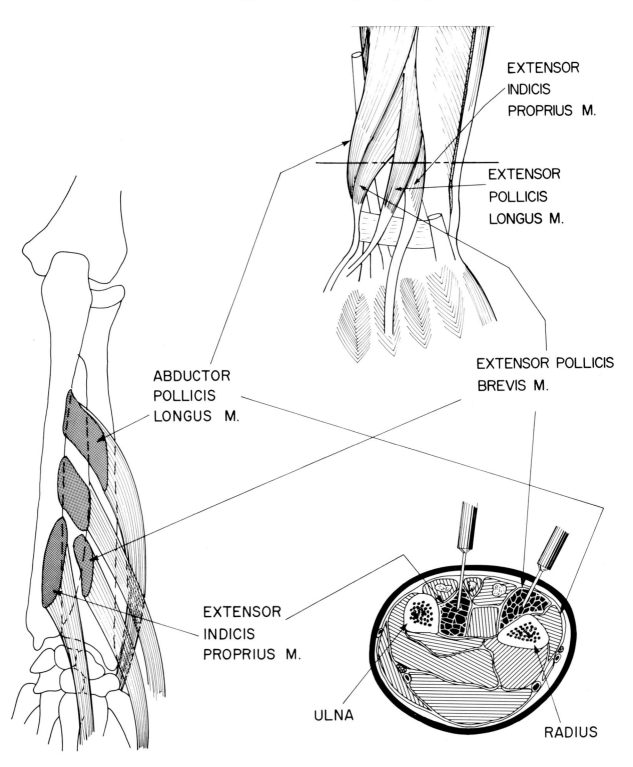

EXTENSOR INDICIS PROPRIUS M.

EXTENSOR POLLICIS LONGUS M.

ABDUCTOR POLLICIS LONGUS M.

EXTENSOR POLLICIS BREVIS M.

EXTENSOR INDICIS PROPRIUS M.

ULNA

RADIUS

III A 19   Extensor pollicis brevis

Nerve Supply: Posterior interosseous N
C_6, C_7

Action: Extension of the first metacarpal and proximal phalanx of the thumb

III A 20   Extensor indicis proprius

Nerve Supply: Posterior interosseous N (the last muscular branch)
C_7, C_8

Action: Extension of the index finger

III A 21   Abductor pollicis longus

Nerve Supply: Posterior interosseous N
C_6, C_7, and (C_8)

Action: Extension, abductor and external rotation of the thumb (draws the thumb out of a position of opposition)

The extensor indicis proprius is widely used in conduction velocity studies of the radial N. It is innervated by the last muscular branch of the posterior interosseous N. The tendon of the extensor carpi ulnaris is identified at the most medial border of the extensor surface approximately 4 cm above the styloid and the electrode is inserted down toward the ulna from the radial side of the ulnaris tendon.

The abductor pollicis longus and the extensor pollicis brevis are also used in conduction velocity studies of the distal radial N, but the recordings are usually made with surface electrodes.

III A 22   ABDUCTOR POLLICIS BREVIS
III A 23   FLEXOR POLLICIS BREVIS
III A 24   OPPONENS POLLICIS

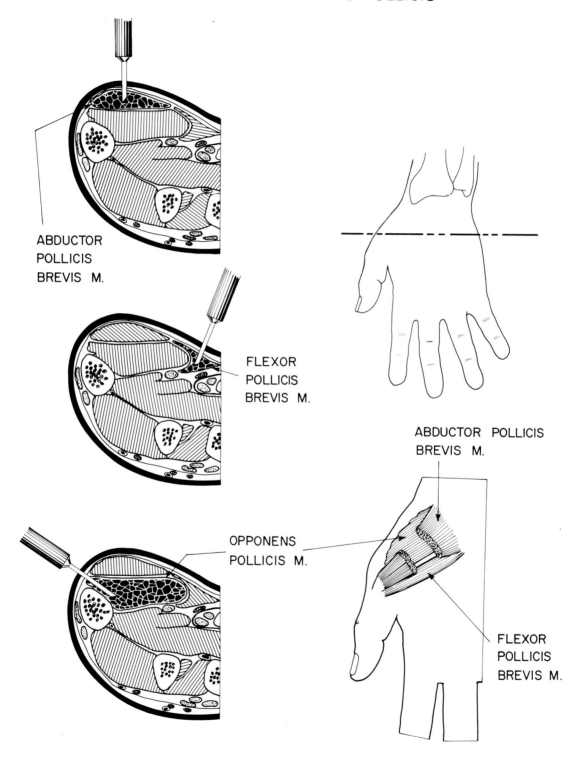

ABDUCTOR
POLLICIS
BREVIS M.

FLEXOR
POLLICIS
BREVIS M.

OPPONENS
POLLICIS M.

ABDUCTOR POLLICIS
BREVIS M.

FLEXOR
POLLICIS
BREVIS M.

III A 22   Abductor pollicis brevis

Nerve Supply: Median N (recurrent branch)
C_8, T_1

Action: Abduction of thumb

III A 23   Flexor pollicis brevis

Nerve Supply: Median N to superficial head
C_8, T_1
Ulnar N to deep head
C_8, T_1

Action: Flexion of the thumb

III A 24   Opponens pollicis

Nerve Supply: Median N
C_8, T_1

Action: Opposition of the thumb

The abductor lies superficially and is the most obvious contributor to the thenar eminence. The medial and lateral margins of the short abductor are easily palpated; the flexor pollicis brevis is located adjacent to the medial edge. The opponens pollicis is a deeper lying muscle which most reliably can be penetrated with the needle electrode along the anterolateral portion of the first metacarpal where the muscle makes its insertion. The depression between the abductor pollicis brevis and the first metacarpal is palpated and the electrode is slid in, anteriorly to the bone.

III A 25   ABDUCTOR DIGITI QUINTI
III A 26   FIRST DORSAL INTEROSSEOUS
III A 27   ADDUCTOR POLLICIS

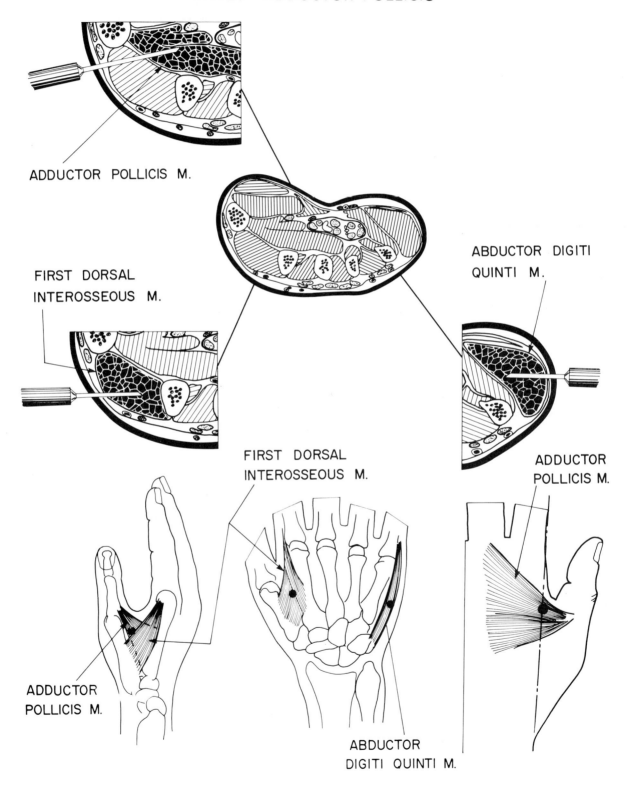

ADDUCTOR POLLICIS M.

FIRST DORSAL
INTEROSSEOUS M.

ABDUCTOR DIGITI
QUINTI M.

FIRST DORSAL
INTEROSSEOUS M.

ADDUCTOR
POLLICIS M.

ADDUCTOR
POLLICIS M.

ABDUCTOR
DIGITI QUINTI M.

III A 25　Abductor digiti quinti

Action:　Abduction of the 5th digit

III A 26　First dorsal interosseous

Action:　Abduction of the index finger

III A 27　Adductor pollicis

Action:　Adduction of the thumb

Nerve Supply:　The innervation of these three muscles is the same: Ulnar N and C_8, T_1

The abductor digiti quinti and the first dorsal interosseous M are examined with relative ease; the needle electrode is inserted for a short distance since both muscles are quite superficial.

The adductor is a deep palmar muscle and can be approached ventrally by insertion of the electrode down into the muscle, along the edge of the flexor pollicis brevis on a line with the radial edge of the index finger or from the dorsal surface at the lateral edge of the first dorsal interosseous, just distal to its juncture with the first metacarpal.

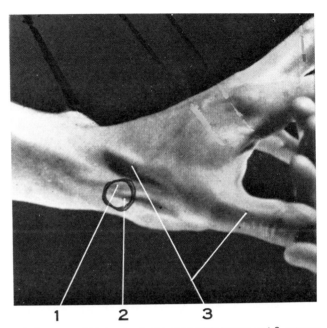

1. Extensor pollicis brevis; *2,* abductor pollicis longus; and *3,* extensor pollicis longus. (Modified from R. D. Lockhart: *Living Anatomy,* Ed. 5, London: Faber and Faber, Ltd., 1959.

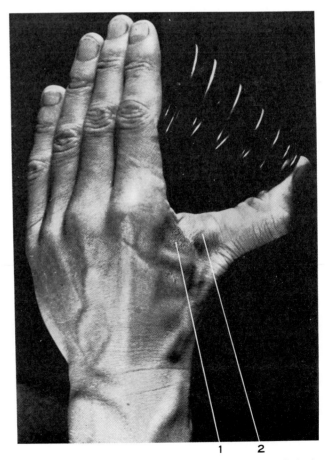

1, First dorsal interosseous and *2,* adductor pollicis. (From R. D. Lockhart: *Living Anatomy,* Ed. 5, London: Faber and Faber, Ltd., 1959.)

III A 28 LUMBRICALES

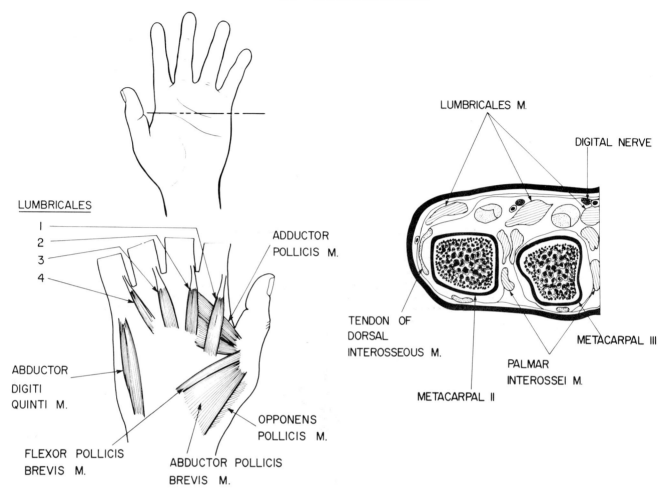

LUMBRICALES

1
2
3
4

ADDUCTOR
POLLICIS M.

ABDUCTOR
DIGITI
QUINTI M.

OPPONENS
POLLICIS M.

FLEXOR POLLICIS
BREVIS M.

ABDUCTOR POLLICIS
BREVIS M.

LUMBRICALES M.

DIGITAL NERVE

TENDON OF
DORSAL
INTEROSSEOUS M.

METACARPAL III

PALMAR
INTEROSSEI M.

METACARPAL II

III A 28   Lumbricales

Nerve Supply: Median N (lateral lumbricalis)
C_8, T_1
Ulnar N (medial lumbricalis)
C_8, T_1

Action: Flexion of metacarpal joints
Extension of interphalangeal joints

There is little need to examine the lumbricales M in clinical electromyography since the integrity of the C_8, T_1 roots or that of the distal median and ulnar nerves may be demonstrated by examining the other intrinsic hand muscles. There is the usual exception—specific identification of a localized lesion such as injury to the deep ulnar nerve incident to fracture of the hamate bone. The lumbricales are entered by penetration from the palmar surface, directing the electrode to approach the radial side of the volar surface of the corresponding metacarpal, II–V. The bellies of the lumbricales are located along the palmar folds as indicated. The first lumbricale is fairly prominent and easily palpated distal to the prominence of the thenar eminence to the radial side of metacarpal II. Accuracy may be enhanced by a voluntary contraction of the long flexor to the digit since the lumbricale originates from the radial side of the long flexor tendons in the palm of the hand.

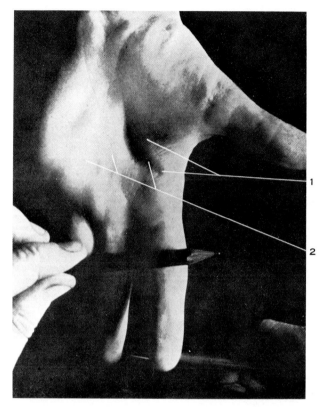

1, First lumbrical M, and 2, position of the long flexor tendons. (From R. D. Lockhart: *Living Anatomy*, Ed. 5, London: Faber and Faber, Ltd., 1959.)

III B 1 BRACHIAL PLEXUS

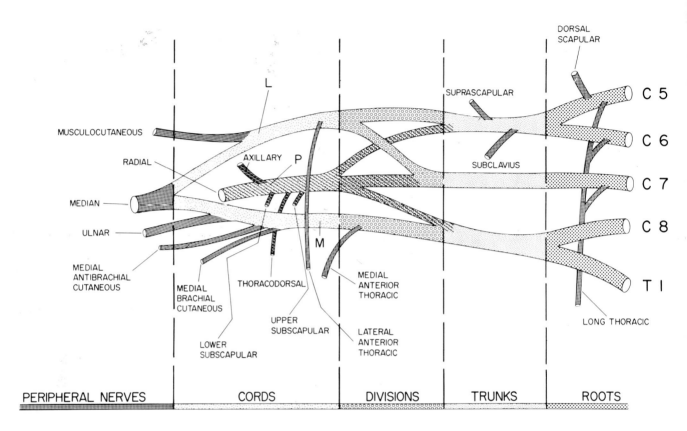

PERIPHERAL NERVES   CORDS   DIVISIONS   TRUNKS   ROOTS

L – LATERAL
M – MEDIAL
P – POSTERIOR

ANTERIOR
POSTERIOR

III B 1   Brachial plexus (diagram)

The brachial plexus is included in this text as one of several "quick" reference diagrams. For example, its study quickly reveals that anterior rami level lesions require examination of the rhomboidii and the serratus anterior. Traumatic involvement at the junction of the C_5–C_6 roots of the upper trunk is frequently identified by examination of the suprascapular distribution. Examination of the coracobrachialis and/or the biceps (musculocutaneous N) and the clavicular portion of the pectoralis major (partially by the lateral anterior thoracic N) will identify paresis due to a lateral cord lesion when the patient's symptoms are clinically most obvious in the median N distribution.

III B 2 BRACHIAL PLEXUS (SUPRACLAVICULAR FOSSA)

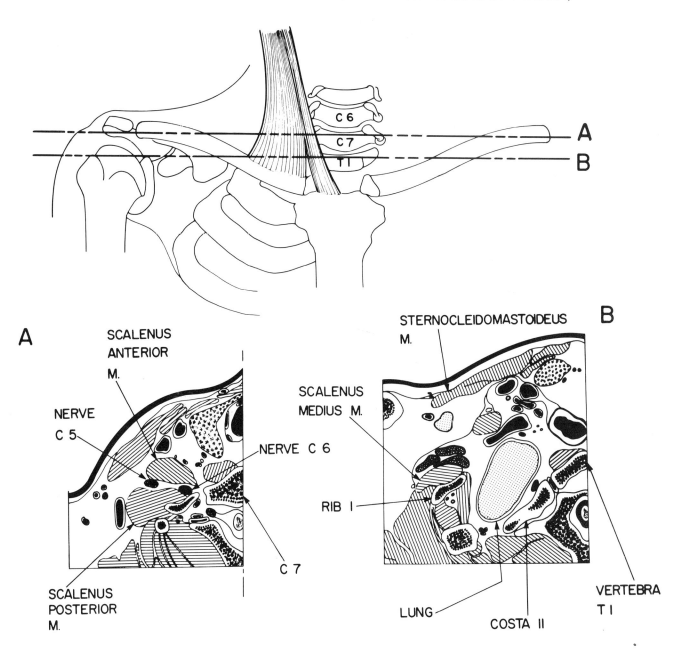

C 6
C 7
T I
A
B

A

SCALENUS
ANTERIOR
M.

NERVE
C 5

NERVE C 6

C 7

SCALENUS
POSTERIOR
M.

STERNOCLEIDOMASTOIDEUS
M.

B

SCALENUS
MEDIUS M.

RIB I

LUNG

COSTA II

VERTEBRA
T I

III B 2   Supraclavicular fossa—brachial plexus

Electrostimulation is carried out at the level of the supraclavicular fossa in evaluation of proximal conduction in the cords and in the most proximal portions of the peripheral nerves of the upper extremity. Two sections are shown, A, at the level of C_6-C_7 and B, through T_1 which intersects Erb's point (the junction of the posterior border of the sternocleidomastoid and the superior margin of the clavicle). Inspection of section A shows that the spinal nerves are still quite distinct and no trunk formation has taken place. It would appear then that stimulation at the lower level through Erb's point is much more appropriate in the study of the formed plexus. Examination of section B in contrast shows the three major trunks have been organized and lie just anterior to the scalenus medius M. The problem of the depth at which the trunks are located and the obvious imprecision of stimulation via the spread of volume conduction makes location of the effective cathode and therefore distance measurement somewhat unreliable.

III B 3   BRACHIAL PLEXUS AND AXILLARY PORTIONS OF MEDIAN, ULNAR AND RADIAL NERVES

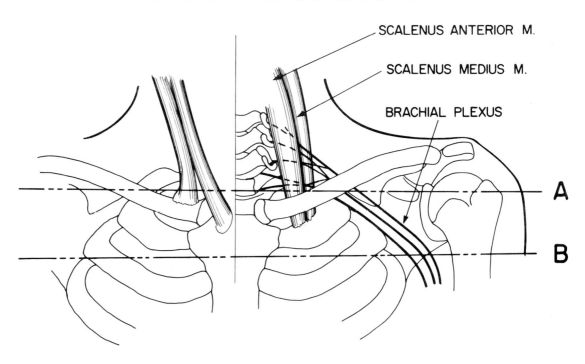

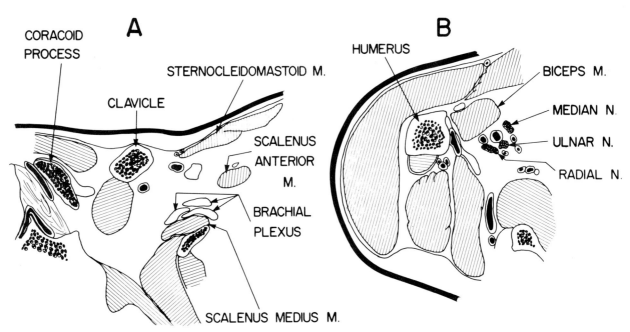

III B 3 **Brachial plexus**
        A. Level at Erb's point
        B. Level through the surgical neck of the humerus

At the level of Erb's point, the cords of the brachial plexus are formed and lie on the scalenus medius and posterior to the scalenus anterior and sterno-cleidomastoid. Because of the depth in position of the plexus and the proximity of each cord to one another, accurate distance measurement in stimulation stud-ies can be quite imaginative. The imprecision is most apparent in radial N studies because the posterior cord is the deepest of all.

In the axilla the neurovascular bundle is just inferior to the coracobrachialis-short head of the bi-ceps muscle mass; the median, ulnar and radial N surround the posteromedial aspect of the brachial artery.

III B 4   MEDIAN NERVE

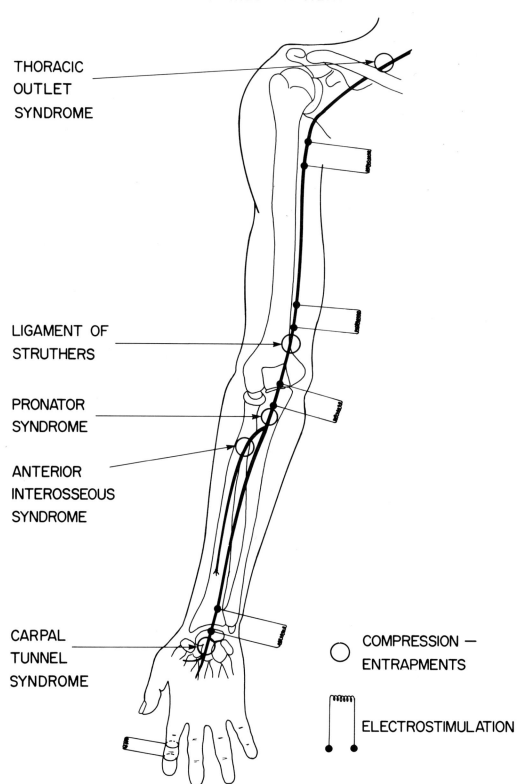

THORACIC
OUTLET
SYNDROME

LIGAMENT OF
STRUTHERS

PRONATOR
SYNDROME

ANTERIOR
INTEROSSEOUS
SYNDROME

CARPAL
TUNNEL
SYNDROME

COMPRESSION —
ENTRAPMENTS

ELECTROSTIMULATION

III B 4 Median N (diagram)

Involvement of the upper trunk or lateral cord of the brachial plexus in the thoracic outlet syndrome is relatively infrequent when compared to the inferior portion of the plexus but nevertheless it may occur when the bony abnormalities are associated with abundant and aberrant fibrous bands. The information regarding the ligament of Struthers is presented on page 64, the anterior interosseous nerve syndrome on page 68, the carpal tunnel on page 88, and the pronator syndrome on page 66.

III B 5   LIGAMENT OF STRUTHERS

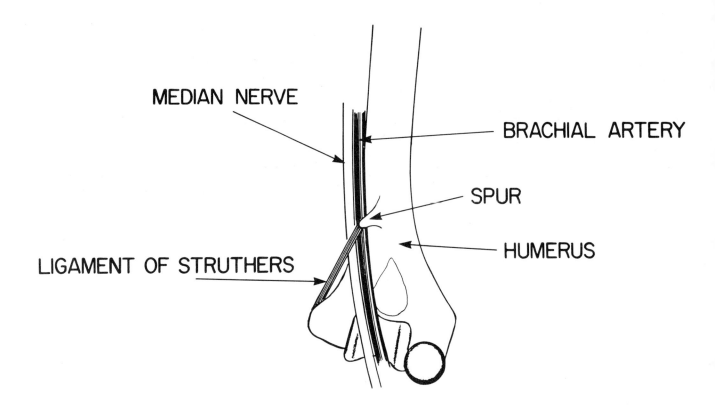

MEDIAN NERVE

BRACHIAL ARTERY

SPUR

HUMERUS

LIGAMENT OF STRUTHERS

III B 5   Ligament of Struthers

The ligament is an anamolous structure which runs from an abnormal spur on the anteromedial aspect of the lower humerus to the medial epicondyle. A fibro-osseous tunnel is formed which may compress the brachial neurovascular bundle to cause vascular, neurological or combined deficit. The presence of this abnormality must be considered in the careful differentiation from more distal entrapments of the median nerve which it grossly resembles, i.e., pronator syndrome or the anterior interosseous syndrome.

III B 6   MEDIAN NERVE—"PRONATOR SYNDROME"

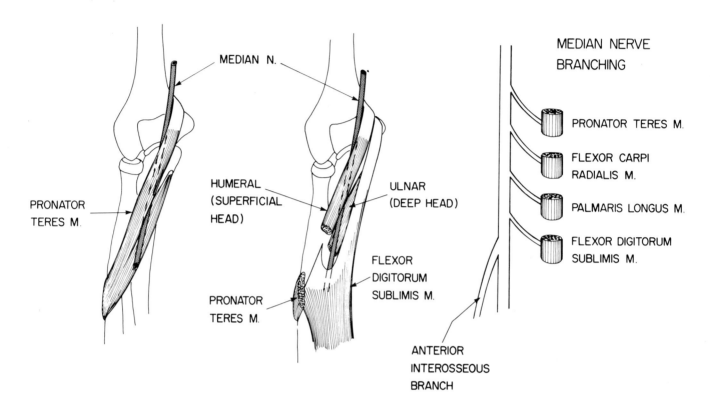

MEDIAN N.

PRONATOR
TERES M.

HUMERAL
(SUPERFICIAL
HEAD)

ULNAR
(DEEP HEAD)

FLEXOR
DIGITORUM
SUBLIMIS M.

PRONATOR
TERES M.

ANTERIOR
INTEROSSEOUS
BRANCH

MEDIAN NERVE
BRANCHING

PRONATOR TERES M.

FLEXOR CARPI
RADIALIS M.

PALMARIS LONGUS M.

FLEXOR DIGITORUM
SUBLIMIS M.

III B 6   Pronator syndrome

The median N comes into the forearm between the superficial and deep heads of the pronator teres. As soon as it passes this point, it dips under the membranous raphe connecting two heads of the flexor digitorum sublimus to run distalward under this digital flexor. The branch from the median N to the pronator arises just proximal to, or at the level of, the two heads of the pronator M. Then, the branches to the flexor carpi radialis, palmaris longus and flexor digitorum sublimus usually come before the anterior interosseous N originates. Therefore, the key to the differential of pronator and anterior interosseous syndrome can be the distribution of electromyographic (EMG) abnormalities. The pronator is spared in the pronator syndrome but the entire median trunk which is distal is affected. In the anterior interosseous N syndrome, the pronator, flexor carpi radialis, palmaris longus, etc., are spared but the anterior interosseous N distribution is affected. In the latter, the sensory distribution of the median is, of course, spared.

III B 7 ANTERIOR OSSEOUS SYNDROME

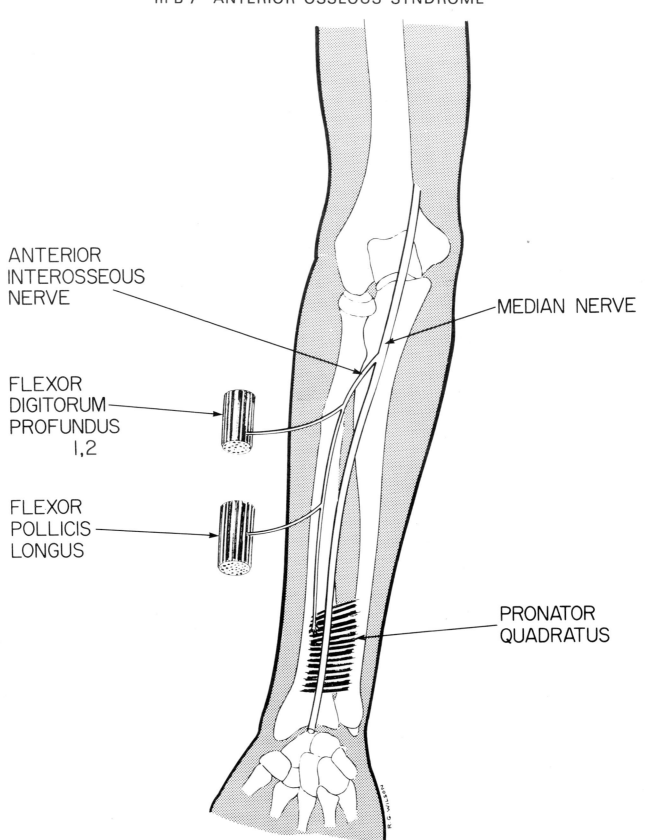

ANTERIOR
INTEROSSEOUS
NERVE

MEDIAN NERVE

FLEXOR
DIGITORUM
PROFUNDUS
1,2

FLEXOR
POLLICIS
LONGUS

PRONATOR
QUADRATUS

III B7   Anterior interosseous syndrome

The anterior interosseous N is purely motor with a usual distribution to the (1) flexor pollicis longus M, (2) radial portion of the flexor digitorum profundus M, and (3) pronator quadratus M.

The nerve rather frequently participates in anomalous distributions, i.e., innervation of all portions of the flexor digitorum profundus, cross-overs (Martin-Gruber communication) to the ulnar nerve, "all median hands," etc.

Compression of the anterior interosseous nerve is a well recognized entity (Kiloh-Nevin syndrome). The etiology involves its vulnerability at its point of origin by such anatomical variations as may concern the tendinous origin of the ulnar head of the pronator teres or of the flexor digitorum sublimus.

III B 8   ULNAR NERVE

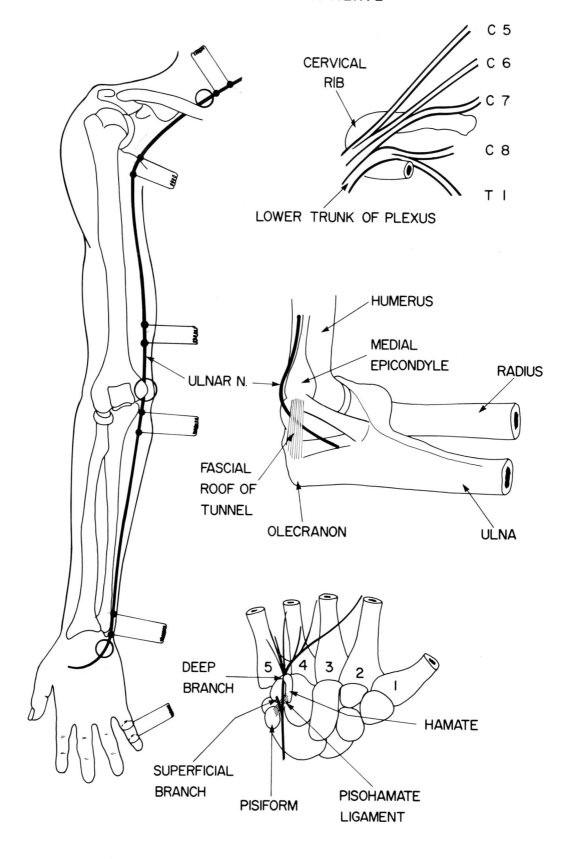

CERVICAL RIB

C 5
C 6
C 7
C 8
T I

LOWER TRUNK OF PLEXUS

HUMERUS

MEDIAL EPICONDYLE

RADIUS

ULNAR N.

FASCIAL ROOF OF TUNNEL

OLECRANON

ULNA

DEEP BRANCH

5 4 3 2 1

HAMATE

SUPERFICIAL BRANCH

PISIFORM

PISOHAMATE LIGAMENT

III B 8   Ulnar N (diagram)

This general view of the ulnar N indicates the "favorite" locations of compressive lesions and the sites of electrostimulation useful in the demonstration of conduction defects.

1. Typical "outlet syndrome" lesion—a cervical rib showing the resultant arching course of the lower trunk of the plexus and its exposure to compression and trauma. The most demonstrable clinical defect which results is manifest in the ulnar nerve, C_8-T_1 distribution.

2. The cubital tunnel is formed at the medial epicondyle of the humerus. Because the innervation to the flexor carpi ulnaris may arise above the epicondylar level, at the epicondylar level or below, the absence or presence of involvement of this muscle may be an unreliable observation in definition of the exact level of the lesion.

3. Guyon's canal—the ulnar tunnel. The specific clinical or electromyographic finding will depend on exactly which part of the distal ulnar N trunk is affected—i.e., if, before bifurcation into superficial and deep branches, a lesion may result in global sensory and motor defect, a lesion just distal to the bifurcation will preserve sensation in the ulnar distribution of the digits but cause motor defects in the ulnar intrinsic muscles with the exception of the palmaris brevis.

III B 9 RADIAL NERVE

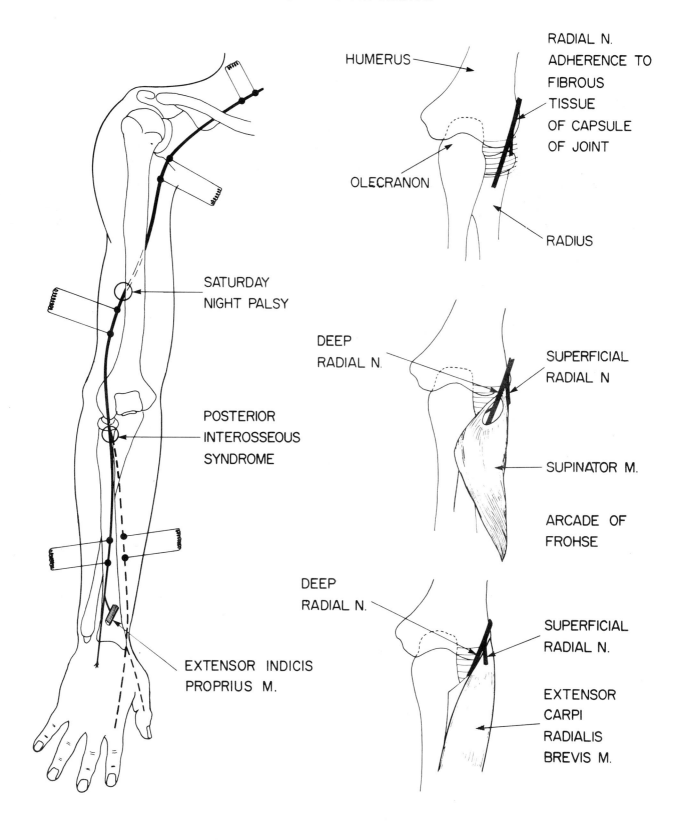

HUMERUS

OLECRANON

RADIAL N.
ADHERENCE TO
FIBROUS
TISSUE
OF CAPSULE
OF JOINT

RADIUS

SATURDAY
NIGHT PALSY

POSTERIOR
INTEROSSEOUS
SYNDROME

EXTENSOR INDICIS
PROPRIUS M.

DEEP
RADIAL N.

SUPERFICIAL
RADIAL N

SUPINATOR M.

ARCADE OF
FROHSE

DEEP
RADIAL N.

SUPERFICIAL
RADIAL N.

EXTENSOR
CARPI
RADIALIS
BREVIS M.

III B 9 Radial N (diagram)

"Saturday night" palsy is the most common pressure neuropathy involving the radial nerve. It is believed to result from prolonged extrinsic compression of the nerve at the position of its penetration through the lateral intermuscular septum. As is well known, the clinical history usually involves excessive intake of alcohol followed by a long period of semi-stuperous sleep.

After the radial nerve passes down into the forearm it bifurcates into its deep and superficial divisions. The deep portion, the posterior interosseous nerve, passes through the supinator muscle to the posterior aspect of the arm where it eventually comes into contact with the interosseous membrane. The posterior interosseous syndrome is a rather complex entity which involves a number of possible anatomical variants and abnormalities.

1. As the radial nerve passes down toward the supinator it passes the radiohumeral joint and is usually loosely tethered to the joint capsule. A firm, constricting band, however, may be present and compress the intact or bifurcated nerve trunk. Under these circumstances, the innervation to the brachioradialis and the extensor carpi radialis muscles remains intact.

2. A short distance distally the nerve dips under the relatively sharp and tough edge of the extensor carpi radialis brevis which may impinge on the nerve, especially during pronation.

3. The point at which the deep radial N enters the supinator M is not a simple slit but is an arch called the arcade of Frohse which may be fibrotendinous and compressive.

4. The posterior interosseous nerve may be compromised within the substance of the supinator mass itself by tumor or vascular anomaly.

Aside from demonstration of a segmental conduction defect, identification of the level of the lesion may be enhanced by the knowledge that the extensor carpi radialis longus is innervated above the bifurcation of the main trunk of the radial N and that the supinator M begins to receive its innervation just before the deep branch penetrates its mass. After the posterior interosseous nerve leaves the supinator it innervates the superficial layer of extensor muscles (extensor digitorum communis, extensor carpi ulnaris, etc.) so that the brachioradialis, extensor carpi radialis, and supinator are spared in the "supinator syndrome" but the extensor digitorum and other distally innervated muscles are affected. The posterior interosseous N then descends on the superficial surfaces of the deep extensor muscles and gives branches into the surface of each of them; the last muscular branch goes to the extensor indicis proprius M, arising about 8 or 10 cm above the ulnar styloid.

III B 10   RADIAL NERVE
LEVEL: APPROX. 7.5 cm BELOW MEDIAL EPICONDYLE

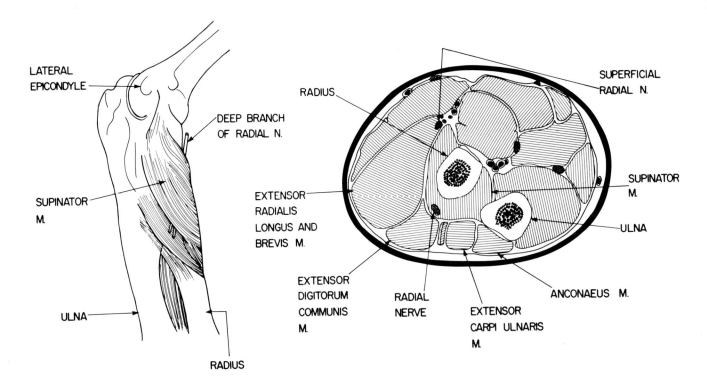

LATERAL
EPICONDYLE

DEEP BRANCH
OF RADIAL N.

SUPINATOR
M.

ULNA

RADIUS

RADIUS

SUPERFICIAL
RADIAL N.

SUPINATOR
M.

ULNA

EXTENSOR
RADIALIS
LONGUS AND
BREVIS M.

EXTENSOR
DIGITORUM
COMMUNIS
M.

RADIAL
NERVE

EXTENSOR
CARPI ULNARIS
M.

ANCONAEUS M.

III B 10   Radial N
Level: about 7.5 cm below the medial
epicondyle

At this cross sectional level the supinator muscle is seen to almost surround the radius. The deep branch of the radial N, the posterior interosseous N, is within the substance of the muscle and the superficial radial N lies in close proximity to the extensor carpi radialis. The frontal section shows the region of penetration of the supinator by the posterior interosseous N and its exit between the two layers of the muscle at its inferior border.

III B 11   SUPERFICIAL RADIAL NERVE
LEVEL: FOREARM

A) 12 cms ABOVE RADIAL STYLOID
B) 9 cms ABOVE RADIAL STYLOID

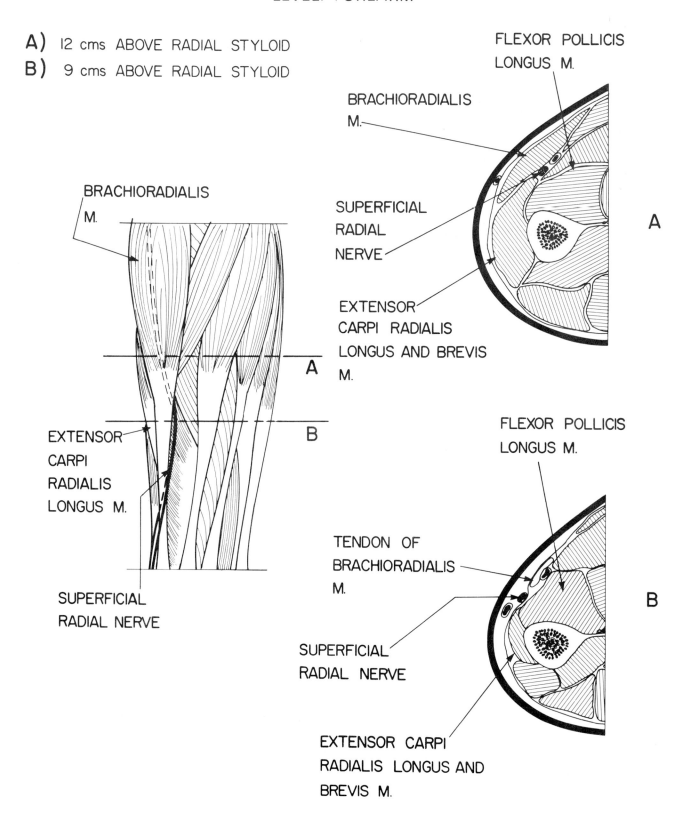

III B 11 Superficial radial N
Level: Forearm

This section through the forearm showing levels about 12 cm (*A*) and 9 cm (*B*) above the radial styloid are presented mainly to review the superficial radial N progression to a more superficial plane. This information is most pertinent to the recording of the nerve action potential of these purely sensory fibers whether by orthodromic (stimulation of radial digital N distribution to the thumb) or antidromically means (stimulation of the superficial radial N near its emergence at the border of the tendon of the brachioradialis). In *A*, the superficial radial N is still deep to the brachioradialis and adjacent to the carpi radial extensors. In *B* (about 3 cm distally), it has taken a superficial position, more suitable for electrostimulation or recording of evoked sensory nerve action potentials.

III B 12 SUPERFICIAL RADIAL NERVE
LEVEL: 5 cm ABOVE RADIAL STYLOID

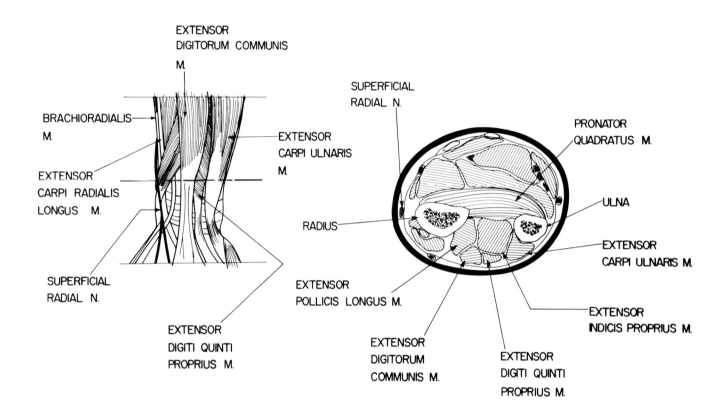

EXTENSOR
DIGITORUM COMMUNIS
M.

BRACHIORADIALIS
M.

EXTENSOR
CARPI RADIALIS
LONGUS M.

SUPERFICIAL
RADIAL N.

EXTENSOR
DIGITI QUINTI
PROPRIUS M.

EXTENSOR
CARPI ULNARIS
M.

SUPERFICIAL
RADIAL N.

PRONATOR
QUADRATUS M.

RADIUS

ULNA

EXTENSOR
CARPI ULNARIS M.

EXTENSOR
POLLICIS LONGUS M.

EXTENSOR
INDICIS PROPRIUS M.

EXTENSOR
DIGITORUM
COMMUNIS M.

EXTENSOR
DIGITI QUINTI
PROPRIUS M.

III B 12   Superficial radial N
Level: Above styloid

This region, about 5 cm above the radial styloid, completes the sequence of study of the superficial radial nerve showing it in a most superficial position and almost precisely located lateral to the radius. A little more distally, as the nerve traverses the anatomical snuff box, it can be palpated by rolling it from side to side against the tendon of the fully contracted extensor pollicis longus.

III B 13 CROSS SECTION AT MID ARM

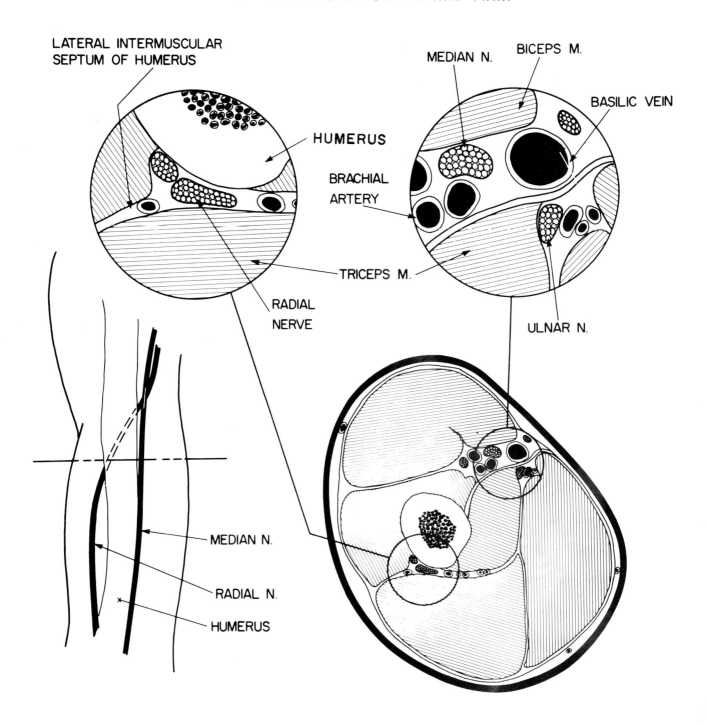

LATERAL INTERMUSCULAR
SEPTUM OF HUMERUS

HUMERUS

TRICEPS M.

RADIAL
NERVE

MEDIAN N.

BICEPS M.

BASILIC VEIN

BRACHIAL
ARTERY

ULNAR N.

MEDIAN N.

RADIAL N.

HUMERUS

III B 13 Upper extremity nerves
Level: Mid-arm cross section

At the mid-arm level, the median N is still located in close relationship to the brachial artery and lies just at the margin of the biceps muscle.

The ulnar N has moved posteriorly to a position inferior to the medial intermuscular septum adjacent to the triceps. The radial N has just about crossed to the lateral side of the arm in the spiral groove so that it is located at the posterolateral edge of the humerus, somewhat inferior to the level of the lateral intermuscular septum. In spite of the fact that there are no really distinct surface marks to differentially locate the median and ulnar, this can be accomplished by the use of minimal intensity stimulating current and careful slow movement of the stimulating electrode. This level does lend itself to exclusion of radial N responses to stimulation of the brachial neurovascular bundle.

III B 14 CROSS SECTION AT EPICONDYLES

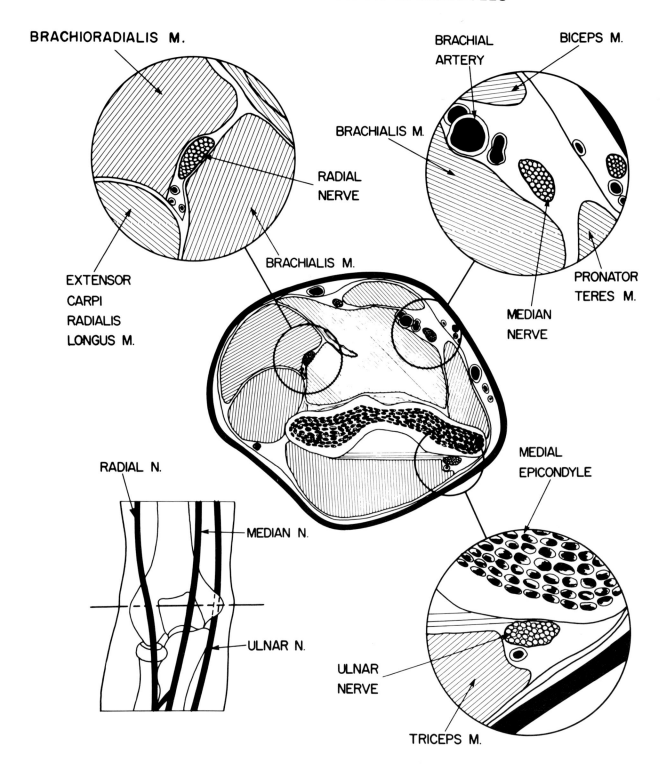

BRACHIORADIALIS M.

BRACHIAL ARTERY

BICEPS M.

BRACHIALIS M.

RADIAL NERVE

EXTENSOR CARPI RADIALIS LONGUS M.

BRACHIALIS M.

PRONATOR TERES M.

MEDIAN NERVE

RADIAL N.

MEDIAN N.

ULNAR N.

MEDIAL EPICONDYLE

ULNAR NERVE

TRICEPS M.

III B 14 Upper extremity nerves
Level: Epicondylar cross section

Median N—maintains its position of proximity to the brachial vessels and again is easily stimulated at the medial margin of the biceps brachii. This position of the nerve makes it vulnerable to injury during deep venipuncture or arterial puncture as well as during cut down procedures, (i.e., by ligature).

Ulnar N—is posterior to the medial epicondyle in the region of the cubital tunnel.

Radial N—the radial N has come through the lateral intermuscular septum and lies between the brachioradialis and brachialis M as it moves distally to pass the elbow joint to enter the forearm. The extensor carpi radialis longus takes its origin at this high level and is located laterally and just inferior to the brachioradialis (useful in study of supinator M entrapment).

III B 15 CROSS SECTION AT MID FOREARM

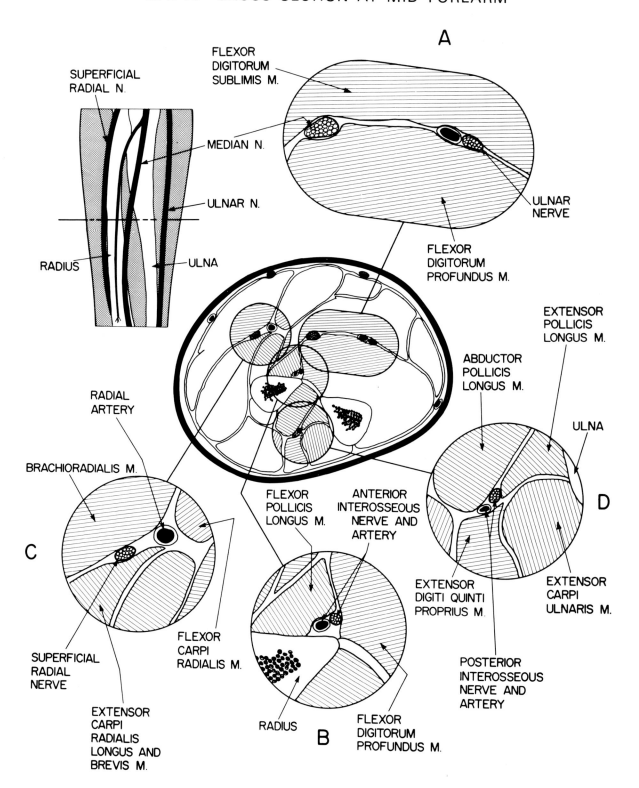

SUPERFICIAL RADIAL N.

FLEXOR DIGITORUM SUBLIMIS M.

MEDIAN N.

ULNAR N.

RADIUS

ULNA

A

ULNAR NERVE

FLEXOR DIGITORUM PROFUNDUS M.

RADIAL ARTERY

BRACHIORADIALIS M.

C

SUPERFICIAL RADIAL NERVE

EXTENSOR CARPI RADIALIS LONGUS AND BREVIS M.

FLEXOR CARPI RADIALIS M.

FLEXOR POLLICIS LONGUS M.

ANTERIOR INTEROSSEOUS NERVE AND ARTERY

RADIUS

B

FLEXOR DIGITORUM PROFUNDUS M.

EXTENSOR DIGITI QUINTI PROPRIUS M.

ABDUCTOR POLLICIS LONGUS M.

EXTENSOR POLLICIS LONGUS M.

ULNA

D

EXTENSOR CARPI ULNARIS M.

POSTERIOR INTEROSSEOUS NERVE AND ARTERY

III B 15 Upper extremity nerves
Level: Mid-forearm cross section

(A) The main trunks of the median and ulnar N make their descent deep in the forearm, in position between flexor digitorum sublimis and flexor digitorum profundus. The median is approximately located along a line from the antecubital fossa to the middle of the wrist and ulnar along a more medially placed line running from just in front of the center of the medial epicondyle to the prominence of pisiform bone.

(B) The anterior interosseous N is located near the membrane on a level with the posterior surfaces of the flexor pollicis longus and the flexor digitorum profundus M.

(C) The superficial radial N runs on the surface of the extensor carpi radialis brevis under the cover of the brachioradialis.

(D) The posterior interosseous N lies deep to the superficial layer of extensor muscles and is typically located on the surface of the abductor pollicis longus M.

III B 16 CROSS SECTION THROUGH RADIAL STYLOID PROCESS

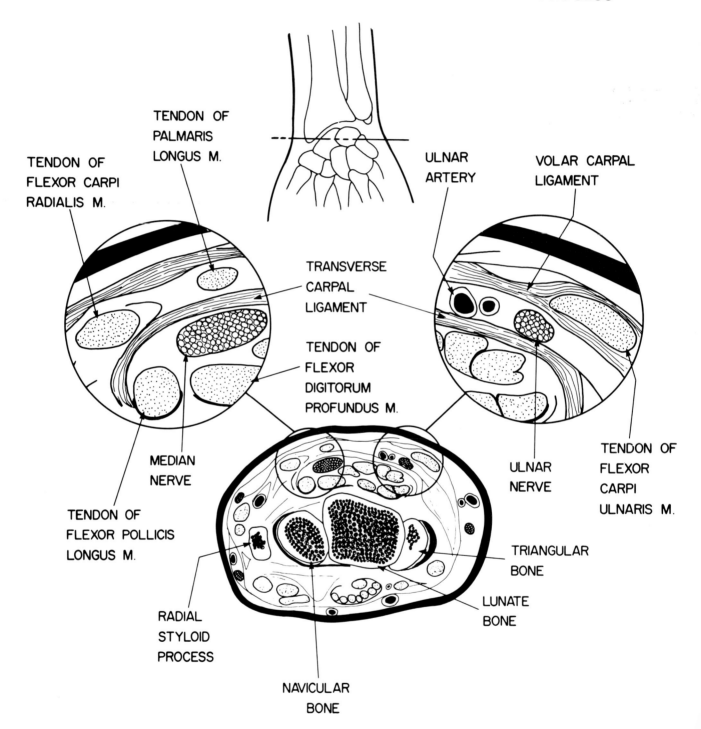

TENDON OF PALMARIS LONGUS M.

TENDON OF FLEXOR CARPI RADIALIS M.

ULNAR ARTERY

VOLAR CARPAL LIGAMENT

TRANSVERSE CARPAL LIGAMENT

TENDON OF FLEXOR DIGITORUM PROFUNDUS M.

MEDIAN NERVE

TENDON OF FLEXOR POLLICIS LONGUS M.

ULNAR NERVE

TENDON OF FLEXOR CARPI ULNARIS M.

TRIANGULAR BONE

LUNATE BONE

RADIAL STYLOID PROCESS

NAVICULAR BONE

III B 16   Upper extremity nerves
Level: Radial styloid cross section

This section is concerned with the respective positions of the median N and ulnar N at the level of the wrist and the relation of each to the transverse carpal ligament.

Median N—is deep to the transverse carpal ligament which has just formed. Just above this point the nerve lies between and deep to the tendons of the flexor carpi radialis and the palmaris longus.

Ulnar N—lies just inferior and slightly lateral to the tendon of the flexor carpi ulnaris. However, it is located superior to the transverse carpal ligament but deep to the superficial volar carpal ligament.

III B 17 CROSS SECTION OF DISTAL CARPAL BONES

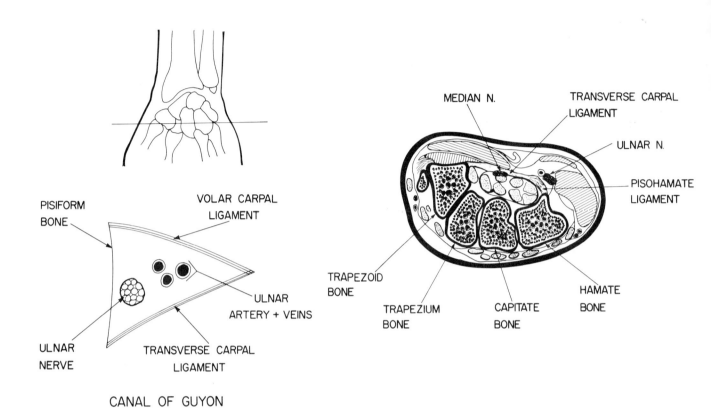

PISIFORM
BONE

VOLAR CARPAL
LIGAMENT

ULNAR
ARTERY + VEINS

ULNAR
NERVE

TRANSVERSE CARPAL
LIGAMENT

CANAL OF GUYON

MEDIAN N.

TRANSVERSE CARPAL
LIGAMENT

ULNAR N.

PISOHAMATE
LIGAMENT

TRAPEZOID
BONE

TRAPEZIUM
BONE

CAPITATE
BONE

HAMATE
BONE

III B 17   Upper extremity nerves
Level: Distal carpal bones

Because of the interest in carpal tunnel disease this cross section of the upper extremity is probably the most familiar one to clinicians. A few pertinent points are worthy of review. The fibro-osseous tunnel is hourglass in shape with the constricted region approximately 2.5 cm from the distal end. The major portion of the tunnel contains the tendons of the four deep flexors and four superficial flexors of the digits, the flexor pollicis longus and the median N, whereas a tiny compartment contains only the tendon of the flexor carpi radialis.

The flexor retinaculum extends distally a considerable distance into the palm with the innervation to the opponens pollicis M turning back and up as a recurrent branch.

The mode of entrance of the ulnar N into the hand is not as widely appreciated as is that of the median. It descends through the "ulnar tunnel" or the canal of Guyon which is a triangular space bounded by the pisiform bone medially, the volar carpal ligament anteriorly and the transverse carpal ligament inferiorly. Just distal to this region, the ulnar nerve divides into its superficial and deep branches. The tunnel continues with the pisohamate ligament as its floor and the palmaris brevis M as its roof. At the hook of the hamate the deep branch makes an abrupt turn and crosses the palm to its ultimate destination, the first dorsal interosseous M.

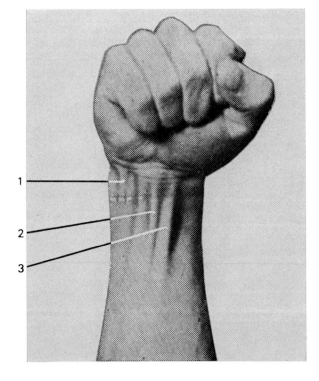

1, Tendon of flexor carpi ulnaris; *2*, palmaris longus; and *3*, flexor carpi radialis. (Modified from R. D. Lockhart: *Living Anatomy*, Ed. 5, London: Faber and Faber, Ltd., 1959.)

III B 18   DIGITAL NERVE

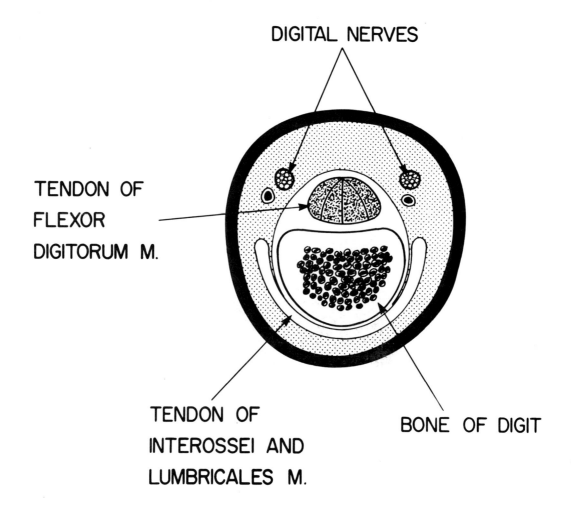

DIGITAL NERVES

TENDON OF
FLEXOR
DIGITORUM M.

TENDON OF
INTEROSSEI AND
LUMBRICALES M.

BONE OF DIGIT

III B 18   Upper extremity nerves
Level: Digital N

The typical distribution to both sides of the flexor digitorum tendon near the palmar surface of the digit is shown. There is a profusion of branching to the palmar surface of the skin but it is well to keep in mind the anterolateral position of the trunks when sensory nerve action potentials are studied. Complete ring electrodes are most suitable for assurance of good contacts.

part IV

TRUNK, PELVIC GIRDLE
and PERINEUM

IV A 1   PARASPINAL MUSCLES—LUMBAR I-II

PSOAS MAJOR M.

QUADRATUS LUMBORUM M.

LONG SPINAL MUSCLES I.E. LONGISSIMUS DORSI M.

SHORT SPINAL MUSCLES I.E. MULTIFIDUS M.

IV A 1 Paraspinal muscles (lumbar I-II)

The general comments concerning segmental nerve distribution in the cervical spine pertain in the lumbar region as well. The technique of insertion into long and short vertebral muscles is also essentially the same; the long muscles in the region may be volitionally activated by extension of the thigh and by a rotary motion of the lumbosacral region. See "Cervical Paravertebral Muscles" (p. 11).

IV A 2   ABDOMINAL MUSCLES: EXTERNAL OBLIQUE, RECTUS ABDOMINUS

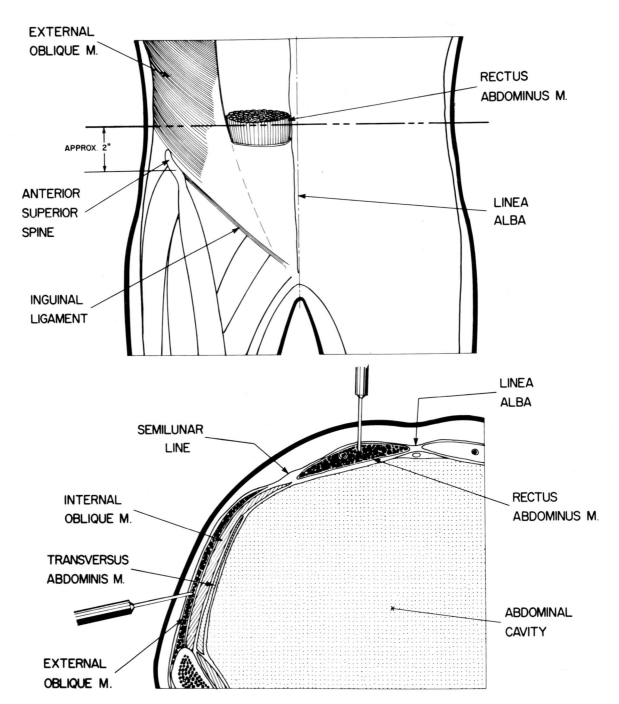

EXTERNAL
OBLIQUE M.

RECTUS
ABDOMINUS M.

APPROX. 2"

ANTERIOR
SUPERIOR
SPINE

LINEA
ALBA

INGUINAL
LIGAMENT

LINEA
ALBA

SEMILUNAR
LINE

INTERNAL
OBLIQUE M.

RECTUS
ABDOMINUS M.

TRANSVERSUS
ABDOMINIS M.

EXTERNAL
OBLIQUE M.

ABDOMINAL
CAVITY

IV A 2 External oblique
Rectus abdominis

Nerve Supply: External oblique: Intercostal N 8–12 and the ilioinguinal and iliohypogastric N

Action: External oblique—both sides act to flex the vertebral column; one side bends and rotates toward the opposite side

Rectus—flexes the column and brings the xiphoid toward the symphesis pubis

The lateral margin of the rectus, the semilunar line, is identified, as are the transverse fibrous bands, the tendinous insertions. The lowest tendinous insertion is at the level of the umbilicus, the highest is at xiphoid level and the third is located in between. The needle is inserted medial to the semilinear line and away from the tendinous insertions.

The external oblique is penetrated on a line with the anterior superior spine but approximately 5 cm superiorly. The electrode is inserted quite superficially in the downward and medial direction of the muscle fibers.

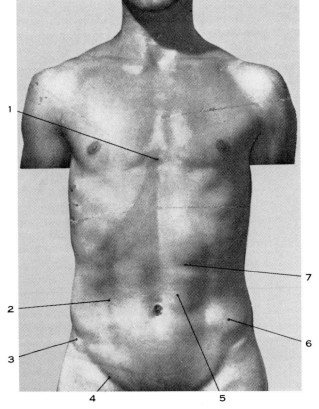

1, Xiphisternal joint; *2*, linea semilunaris; *3*, anterior superior spine; *4*, inguinal ligament; *5*, rectus abdominus; *6*, extensor oblique M; and *7*, tendinous insertion (intersection). (From W. J. Hamilton, G. Simon, and S. G. Ian Hamilton: *Surface and Radiological Anatomy for Students and General Practitioners*, Ed. 5, Cambridge, England; W. Heffer and Sons Ltd., 1971.)

IV A 3 SPHINCTER ANI EXTERNUS MUSCLE

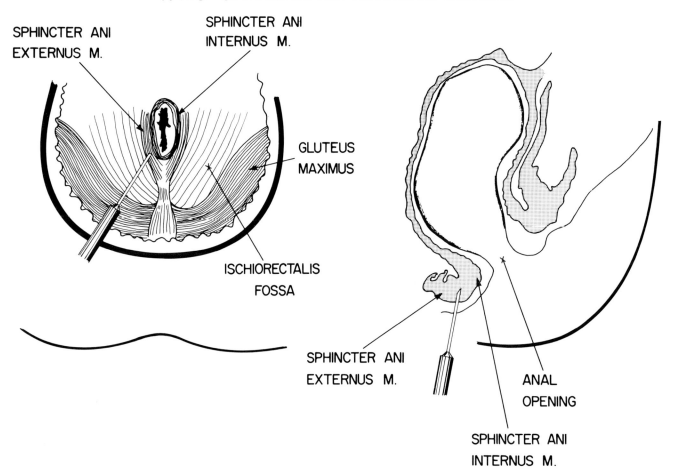

SPHINCTER ANI
EXTERNUS M.

SPHINCTER ANI
INTERNUS M.

GLUTEUS
MAXIMUS

ISCHIORECTALIS
FOSSA

SPHINCTER ANI
EXTERNUS M.

ANAL
OPENING

SPHINCTER ANI
INTERNUS M.

IV A 3   Sphincter ani externus

Nerve Supply: Inferior hemorrhoidal branch
of the pudendal N and S_4

Action: Tonically contracts to keep the anal
orifice closed

The sphincter is a very superficial muscle and is adherent to the perianal skin. The more superficial portion runs from the coccyx to the anus, whereas the deeper portion's fibers surround the anal canal. The recommended technique is to gently introduce a lubricated finger into the anal orifice and then insert the electrode into the muscle using the digit as a guide to prevent penetration through the mucous membrane. Through and through penetration may invite formation of a subsequent ischiorectal abscess.

part V

LOWER EXTREMITY

V A 1   ILIOPSOAS

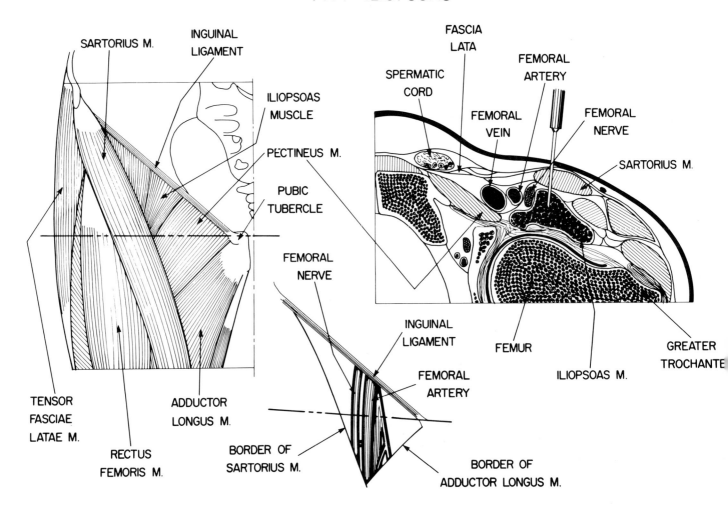

V A 1   Iliopsoas

Nerve Supply: L₂, L₃, and L₄

Action: Flexion of thigh

It is safe to examine the Iliopsoas below the inguinal ligament where the conjoined muscle forms part of the floor of the femoral triangle as shown in the frontal section and the small insert. Needle electrode insertion is carried out on a line between the pubic tubercle and greater trochanter. The femoral artery is identified by palpation as is the medial edge of the sartorius M. The electrode is inserted perpendicularly down into the iliopsoas M which lies just anterior to the ileopectineal bursa and the joint capsule. It is well to insert the needle approximately 2 or 3 cm lateral to the position of the femoral pulse so as to avoid striking the femoral N.

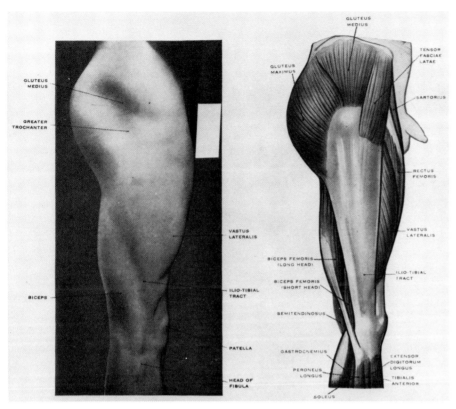

GLUTEUS MEDIUS

GREATER TROCHANTER

VASTUS LATERALIS

ILIO-TIBIAL TRACT

BICEPS

PATELLA

HEAD OF FIBULA

GLUTEUS MEDIUS

GLUTEUS MAXIMUS

TENSOR FASCIAE LATAE

SARTORIUS

RECTUS FEMORIS

VASTUS LATERALIS

BICEPS FEMORIS (LONG HEAD)

BICEPS FEMORIS (SHORT HEAD)

ILIO-TIBIAL TRACT

SEMITENDINOSUS

GASTROCNEMIUS

PERONEUS LONGUS

SOLEUS

EXTENSOR DIGITORUM LONGUS

TIBIALIS ANTERIOR

(From W. J. Hamilton, G. Simon, and S. G. Ian Hamilton: *Surface and Radiological Anatomy for Students and General Practitioners;* Ed. 5, Cambridge, England: W. Heffer and Sons Ltd., 1971.)

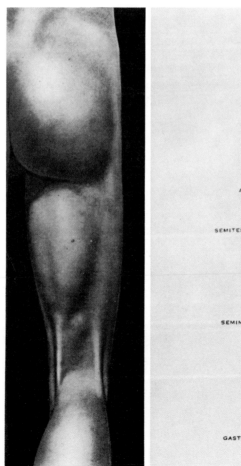

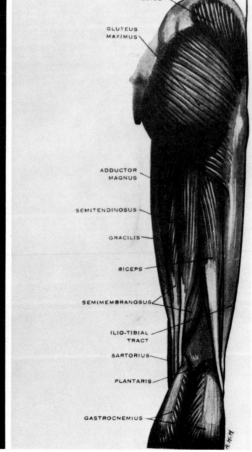

GLUTEUS MEDIUS

GLUTEUS MAXIMUS

ADDUCTOR MAGNUS

SEMITENDINOSUS

GRACILIS

BICEPS

SEMIMEMBRANOSUS

ILIO-TIBIAL TRACT

SARTORIUS

PLANTARIS

GASTROCNEMIUS

(From W. J. Hamilton, G. Simon, and S. G. Ian Hamilton. *Surface and Radiological Anatomy for Students and General Practitioners*, Ed. 5, Cambridge, England: W. Heffer and Sons Ltd., 1971.)

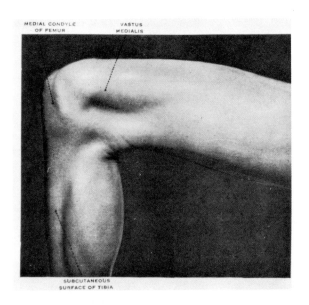

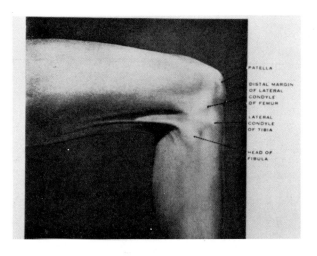

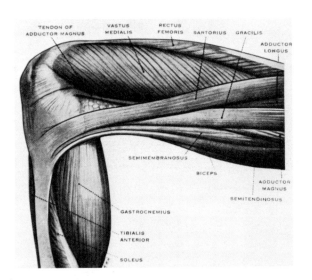

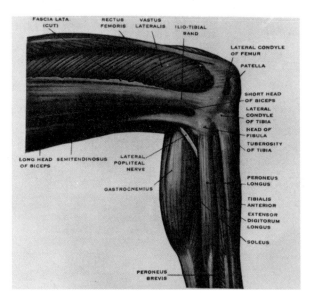

(From W. J. Hamilton, G. Simon, and S. G. Ian Hamilton: *Surface and Radiological Anatomy for Students and General Practitioners*, Ed. 5, Cambridge, England: W. Heffer and Sons Ltd., 1971.)

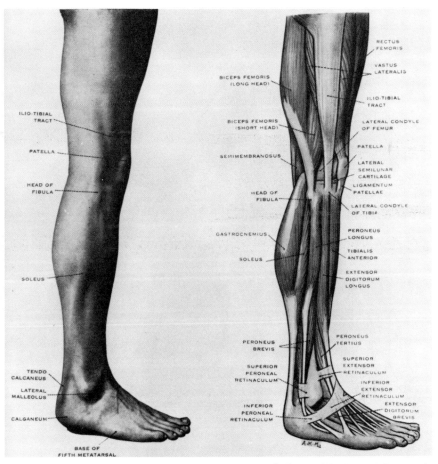

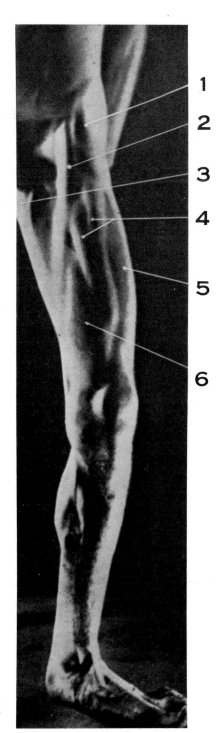

(From W. J. Hamilton, G. Simon, and S. G. Ian Hamilton: *Surface and Radiological Anatomy for Students and General Practitioners*, Ed. 5, Cambridge, England: W. Heffer and Sons Ltd., 1971.)

1, Tensor fascia lata; *2*, sartorius; *3*, adductors; *4*, rectus femoris; *5*, vastus lateralis; and *6*, vastus medialis. (From R. D. Lockhart: *Living Anatomy*, Ed. 5, London: Faber and Faber Ltd., 1959.)

V A 2   TENSOR FASCIAE LATAE

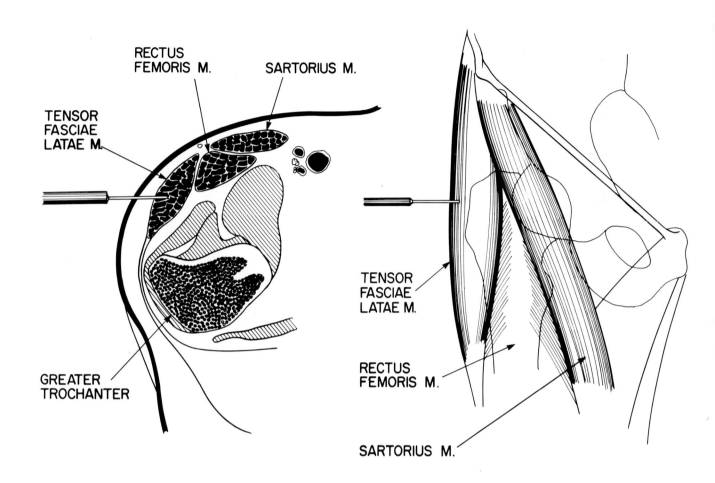

RECTUS
FEMORIS M.

SARTORIUS M.

TENSOR
FASCIAE
LATAE M.

GREATER
TROCHANTER

TENSOR
FASCIAE
LATAE M.

RECTUS
FEMORIS M.

SARTORIUS M.

V A 2 Tensor fasciae latae

Nerve Supply: Superior gluteal N
L_4, L_5, and S_1

Action: Flexion and internal rotation of the thigh

Electrode insertion is made at the intersection of a line drawn downward from the anterosuperior spine just in front of the greater trochanter to intercept the horizontal plane through the middle of the greater trochanter itself.

V A 3   GLUTEUS MAXIMUS AND GLUTEUS MEDIUS

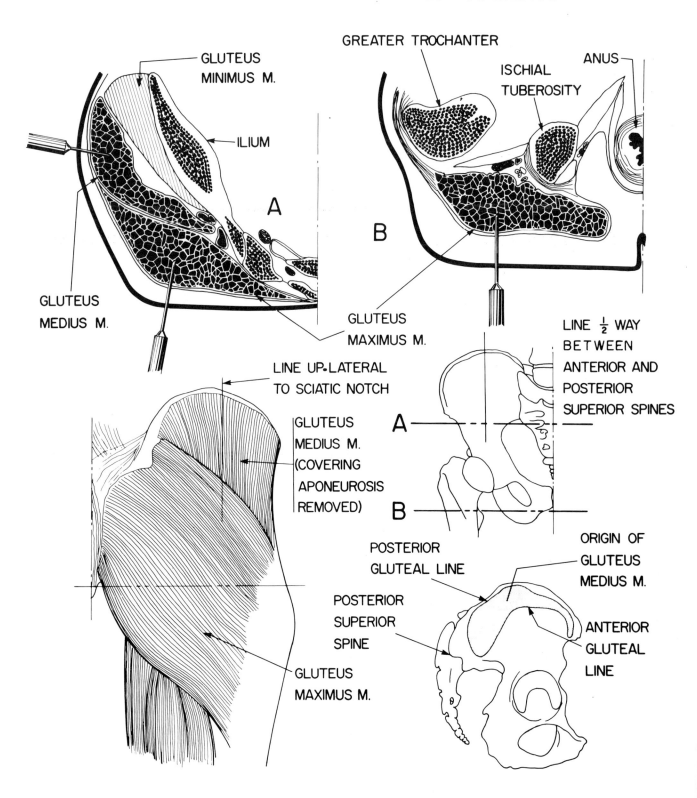

GLUTEUS MINIMUS M.

ILIUM

GLUTEUS MEDIUS M.

A

GREATER TROCHANTER

ISCHIAL TUBEROSITY

ANUS

B

GLUTEUS MAXIMUS M.

LINE UP-LATERAL TO SCIATIC NOTCH

GLUTEUS MEDIUS M. (COVERING APONEUROSIS REMOVED)

GLUTEUS MAXIMUS M.

LINE ½ WAY BETWEEN ANTERIOR AND POSTERIOR SUPERIOR SPINES

A

B

POSTERIOR GLUTEAL LINE

POSTERIOR SUPERIOR SPINE

ORIGIN OF GLUTEUS MEDIUS M.

ANTERIOR GLUTEAL LINE

V A 3 Gluteus maximus

Nerve Supply: Inferior gluteal N
L_5, S_1, and S_2

Action: Extension of the hip joint

Gluteus medius

Nerve Supply: Superior gluteal N.
L_4, L_5, and S_1

Action: Abduction of the thigh

The gluteus maximus covers most of the buttock while the gluteus medius is located superior to the upper margin of the maximus. The needle electrode is inserted into the maximus one-third from the lateral edge, on a line from the upper border of the greater trochanter of the femur to the ischial tuberosity.

The medius is examined at a somewhat higher level. The anterior and posterior superior spines are palpated and a vertical line drawn midway. This intersect is located lateral to the sciatic notch so as to avoid the sciatic N. The needle electrode is introduced on this line approximately 5 cm below the crest of the ileum. The origin of the gluteus medius from the ilium is shown in the insert diagram as a matter of reference.

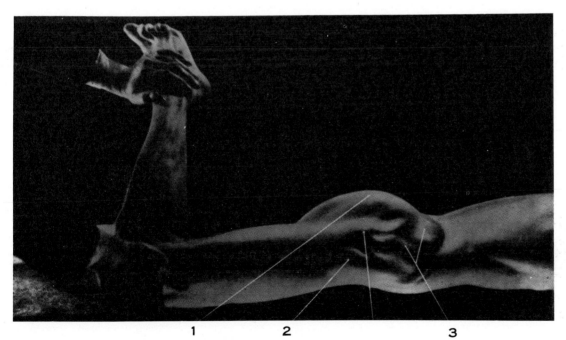

1, Gluteus maximus; 2, tensor fasciae latae; and 3, gluteus medius. (From R. D. Lockhart: *Living Anatomy*, Ed. 5, London: Faber and Faber Ltd., 1959.)

V A 4   SHORT HEAD OF BICEPS

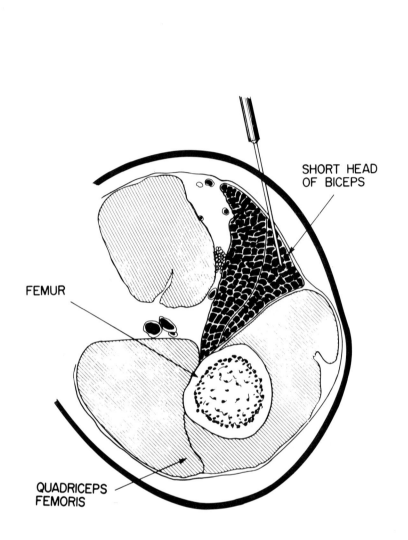

SHORT HEAD
OF BICEPS

FEMUR

QUADRICEPS
FEMORIS

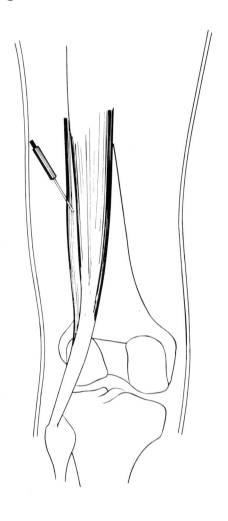

V A 4 Biceps femoris
Short head

Nerve Supply: Sciatic N (peroneal portion)
L_5, S_1, and S_2

Action: Flexion of knee

The tendon of the biceps femoris as it passes over the posterolateral aspect of the knee joint is easily identified. The electrode is inserted at the lateral border of the tendon approximately 12 to 15 cm above the insertion into the fibula. When the tip strikes the femur, the electrode is withdrawn 1 cm or so to lie in the short head of the biceps.

This muscle is a particularly useful one to examine in differentiating peroneal nerve from segmental (L_5) lesions because of its distinct innervation through the peroneal portion of the sciatic nerve before the peroneal becomes an independent structure and in establishing the level of a lesion in the peroneal trunk itself.

V A 5   HAMSTRING MUSCLE
V A 6   ADDUCTOR
V A 7   SARTORIUS
V A 8   QUADRICEPS FEMORIS

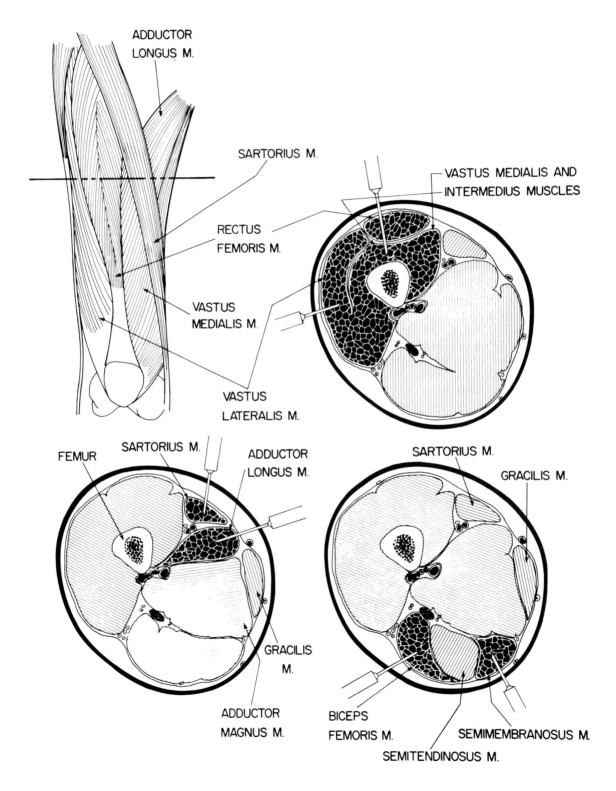

V A 5   Hamstring

Nerve Supply: Sciatic N
L$_5$, S$_1$, and S$_2$

Action: Extension of the thigh
Flexion of the knee

V A 6   Adductor

Nerve Supply: Obturator N
L$_2$, L$_3$, and L$_4$

Action: Adduction of the thigh

V A 7   Sartorius

Nerve Supply: Femoral N
L$_2$, L$_3$

Action: Flexion, external rotation and abduction of the thigh

V A 8   Quadriceps femoris

Nerve Supply: Femoral N
L$_2$, L$_3$, and L$_4$

Action: Extension of leg on the thigh

The cross section which is shown is at the same level for each muscle and is at the junction of the upper one-third and lower two-thirds of the thigh about 23 cm above the upper border of the patella (adult). The straplike sartorius is superficial and runs obliquely across the thigh on a line from the anterosuperior spine to the medial aspect of thigh at about a junction of upper three-fourths and lower one-fourth. At this same level, the vastus medialis is penetrated at a deeper level adjacent to the femur and the vastus lateralis is easily entered from the lateral surface of the thigh. The adductor longus is located medially just inferior to the sartorius. It can be lined up with the prominent adductor tubercle of the pubis.

At this level of the thigh the lateral and medial hamstrings are prominent muscular masses easily identified in a topographical view of the posterior aspect of the thigh. Electrodes are directly inserted into each muscle mass, respectively.

The vastus medialis is very prominent in the lower one-third of the thigh. The electrode can be inserted medial to the edge of the rectus.

V A 9   TIBIALIS ANTERIOR
V A 10   EXTENSOR DIGITORUM LONGUS
V A 11   PERONEUS LONGUS AND BREVIS

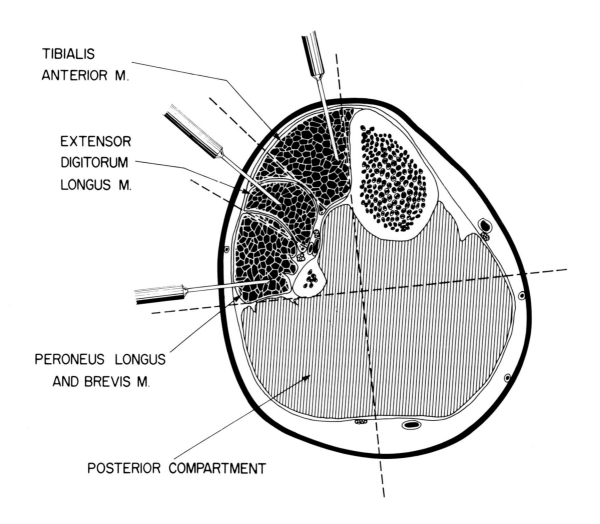

TIBIALIS
ANTERIOR M.

EXTENSOR
DIGITORUM
LONGUS M.

PERONEUS LONGUS
AND BREVIS M.

POSTERIOR COMPARTMENT

V A 9   Tibialis anterior

Nerve Supply: Peroneal N—deep branch
L_4, L_5, and S_1

Action: Dorsi flexion of the foot
Inversion of the foot

V A 10   Extensor digitorum longus

Nerve Supply: Peroneal N—deep branch
L_4, L_5, and S_1

Action: Dorsi flexion of foot
Extension of proximal phalanges of
the four lesser toes

V A 11   Peroneus

Nerve Supply: Peroneal N—superfical branch
L_5, S_1

Action: Eversion of the foot
Plantar flexion of the foot

In the upper half of the leg, the combined anterior and lateral compartments can be roughly divided into three regions extending from the crest of the tibia to the posterior edge of the fibula. The tibialis anterior M is located in the medial third, the peroneus is lined up laterally with the fibula and the middle third is occupied by the extensor digitorum longus.

V A 12   EXTENSOR HALLUCIS LONGUS

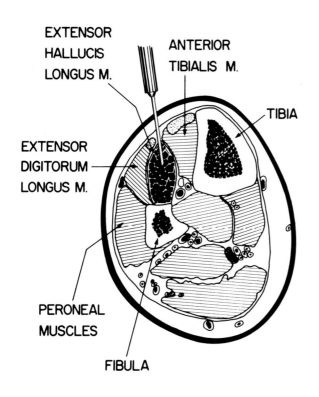

EXTENSOR HALLUCIS LONGUS M.

ANTERIOR TIBIALIS M.

TIBIA

EXTENSOR DIGITORUM LONGUS M.

PERONEAL MUSCLES

FIBULA

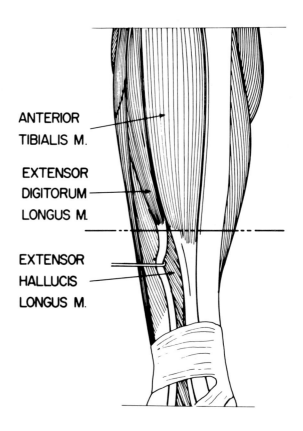

ANTERIOR TIBIALIS M.

EXTENSOR DIGITORUM LONGUS M.

EXTENSOR HALLUCIS LONGUS M.

V A 12   Extensor hallucis longus

Nerve Supply: Peroneal N—deep branch
L₄, L₅, and S₁

Action: Extensor of first toe

At the recommended level for needle electrode insertion, approximately 12 cm above the lateral malleolus, the extensor hallucis longus is practically covered by the distal parts of the anterior tibial muscle and the extensor digitorum longus. The lateral and medial edge of these muscles which are almost completely tendinous are respectively identified and the electrode is inserted between them down to the extensor hallucis.

V A 13 POPLITEUS

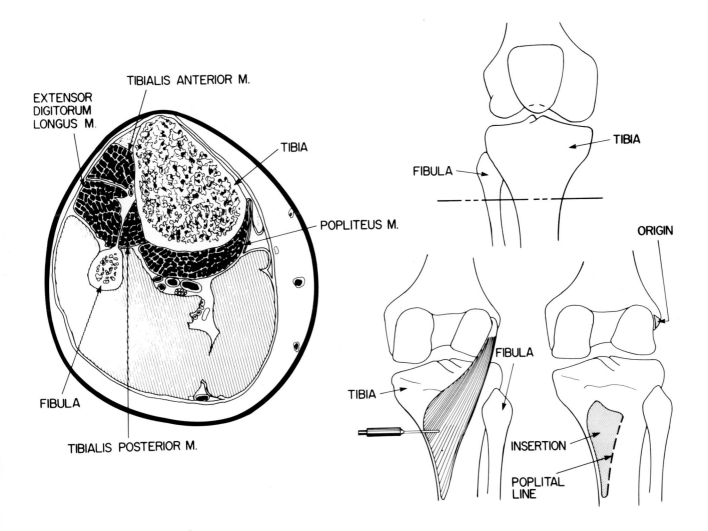

EXTENSOR DIGITORUM LONGUS M.

TIBIALIS ANTERIOR M.

TIBIA

POPLITEUS M.

FIBULA

TIBIALIS POSTERIOR M.

TIBIA

FIBULA

ORIGIN

FIBULA

TIBIA

INSERTION

POPLITAL LINE

V A 13   Popliteus

Nerve Supply: Tibial N
L₄ L₅, and S₁

Action: Flexion and medial rotation of leg (or lateral rotation of femur)

The muscle is deeply located to form the lower part of the floor of the popliteal space. A horizontal line across the level of the neck of the fibula is a landmark. The medial edge of the tibia is palpated and insertion is made at this intersect in the anterolateral direction to the posterior tibial surface. The needle is withdrawn slightly to the belly of the muscle.

Note: Other muscles of the tibial and L₅, S₁ distribution are easier to examine electromyographically. In studies of sciatic nerve conduction, however, it has been noted that recording the motor response from such a large volume muscle as the gastrocnemius may involve considerable error in latency measurement. Needle electrode recording from the popliteus can be used to obviate this possible erroneous factor.

V A 14 GASTROCNEMIUS AND SOLEUS

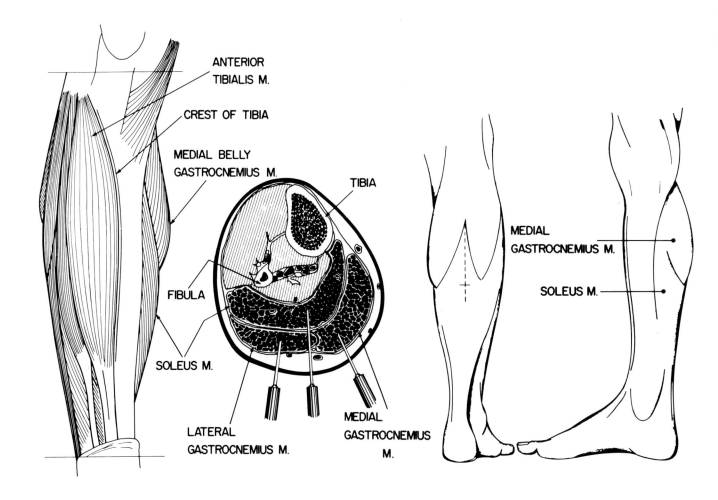

ANTERIOR TIBIALIS M.

CREST OF TIBIA

MEDIAL BELLY GASTROCNEMIUS M.

FIBULA

SOLEUS M.

LATERAL GASTROCNEMIUS M.

TIBIA

MEDIAL GASTROCNEMIUS M.

MEDIAL GASTROCNEMIUS M.

SOLEUS M.

V A 14   **Gastrocnemius**
            Soleus
            Triceps surae

Nerve Supply: Tibial N
                S_1, S_2

Action: Plantar flexion of foot. (Because of its femoral origins, the gastrocnemius is placed at a disadvantage when the knee is flexed.)
Flexion of knee

The landmarks for needle electrode examination are defined by the intersecting lines drawn through the raphe between the lateral and medial bellies of the gastrocnemius as well as the lower edge of these bellies. The lateral and medial gastrocnemius are examined by needle insertion into their respective muscular masses and the soleus is examined by a deeper insertion at the point of intersection of the guidelines. Observation of the frontal view also shows that the soleus is prominent on the posteromedial aspect of the leg just below the easily defined rounded contour of the medial gastrocnemius.

VA 15   ABDUCTOR HALLUCIS
VA 16   ABDUCTOR DIGITI QUINTI
VA 17   FLEXOR DIGITORUM BREVIS

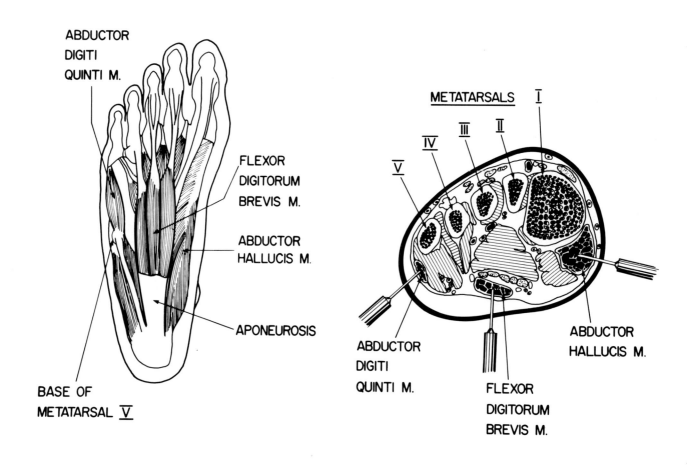

ABDUCTOR
DIGITI
QUINTI M.

FLEXOR
DIGITORUM
BREVIS M.

ABDUCTOR
HALLUCIS M.

APONEUROSIS

BASE OF
METATARSAL V

METATARSALS   I
                        II
                   III
              IV
         V

ABDUCTOR
DIGITI
QUINTI M.

FLEXOR
DIGITORUM
BREVIS M.

ABDUCTOR
HALLUCIS M.

V A 15   Abductor hallucis

Nerve Supply: Medial plantar N
L_5, S_1

Action: Plantar flexes the first toe

V A 16   Abductor digiti quinti

Nerve Supply: Lateral plantar N
S_1, S_2

Action: Abducts the little toe

V A 17   Flexor digitorum brevis

Nerve Supply: Medial plantar N
L_5, S_1

Action: Flexes the middle phalanges of the second to fifth toe

These three form the superficial layer of muscles of the sole. The abductor hallucis runs along the medial border of the foot, the flexor digitorum is in the middle compartment and the abductor digiti quinti is located on the lateral side. For introduction of the needle electrode into these muscles, the prominent head of the fifth metatarsal bone is a good and easily identified landmark. The abductor digitis quinti is penetrated approximately 2 or 3 cm anterior to the bone from a lateral and ventral approach. The flexor digitorum is entered directly on a line, level with the base of the metatarsal. The abductor hallucis is also examined at this same level with the electrode going in a dorsal and medial direction toward the first metatarsal.

V A 18   EXTENSOR DIGITORUM BREVIS

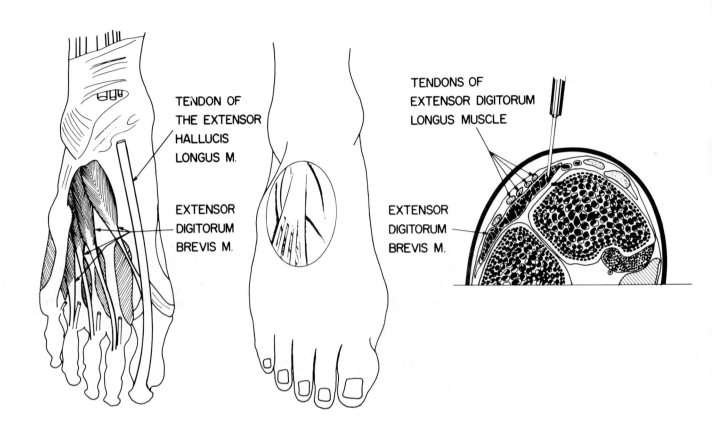

TENDON OF
THE EXTENSOR
HALLUCIS
LONGUS M.

EXTENSOR
DIGITORUM
BREVIS M.

TENDONS OF
EXTENSOR DIGITORUM
LONGUS MUSCLE

EXTENSOR
DIGITORUM
BREVIS M.

V A 18   Extensor digitorum brevis

Nerve Supply: Deep peroneal N
L_5, S_1

Action: Extension of the toes mainly at the metatarsophalangeal joints

The flat extensor digitorum brevis is located on the lateral side of the proximal part of the dorsum of the foot. It is a superficial muscle which is easily palpated and can be seen as a well circumscribed bulge when the toes are extended. Needle electrode insertion is relatively superficial since it is not difficult to penetrate the muscle belly entirely and to strike the underlying metacarpal bone (cuboid).

V A 19   TIBIALIS POSTERIOR

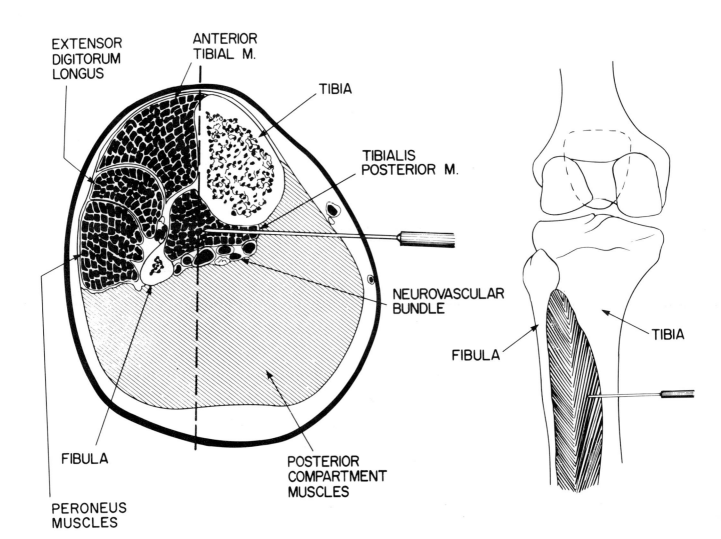

V A 19   Tibialis posterior

Nerve Supply: Posterior tibial N
L₅, S₁

Action: Plantar flexion inversion and abduction of the foot

The following landmarks are used to localize this deep muscle:

1. Medial border of tibia.
2. Horizontal plane—line drawn approximately 10 cm below the prominence of the fibular head.
3. Approximately 2.5 cm posterior to the edge of the tibia at the margin of the medial belly of the gastrocnemius, the electrode is introduced in a lateral and slightly anterior direction to slide along the posterior margin of the tibia until the tip of the electrode is approximately lined up with the medial border of the tibia (the crest).

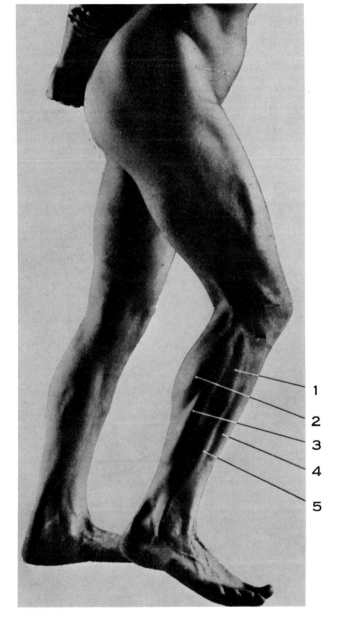

1, Peroneus longus; *2*, gastrocnemius; *3*, soleus; *4*, extensor digitorum longus; and *5*, peroneus brevis. (From R. D. Lockhart: *Living Anatomy*, Ed. 5, London: Faber and Faber, Ltd., 1959.)

V B 1   SACRAL AND COCCYGEAL PLEXUSES

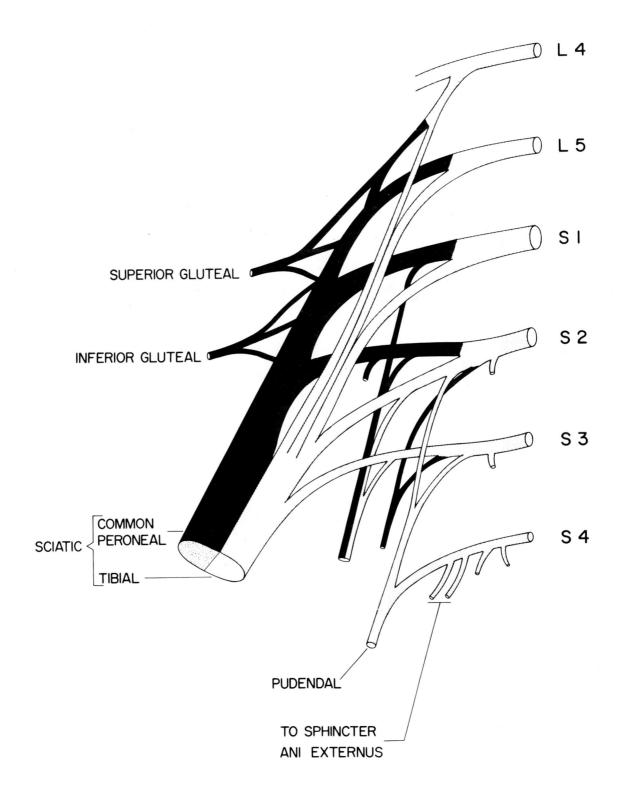

V B 1   Sacral plexus (diagram)

The sacral plexus and lumbosacral diagrams are included in this text for reasons of completeness and ease of referral. The composition of the lateral (common peroneal) and the medial (tibial) portions which contribute to the formation of the sciatic N are emphasized by the difference in hatching and shading. The common roots shared by the sciatic N and the gluteal N are quite obvious and, of course, relate to the definition of a plexus vs. a peripheral nerve lesion. The distribution of S_4 to the innervation of the sphincter ani externis is also prominently displayed since it represents the simplest means of examination of these most caudad roots.

V B 2   SCIATIC NERVE

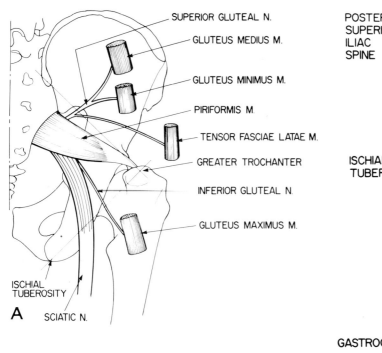

SUPERIOR GLUTEAL N.

GLUTEUS MEDIUS M.

GLUTEUS MINIMUS M.

PIRIFORMIS M.

TENSOR FASCIAE LATAE M.

GREATER TROCHANTER

INFERIOR GLUTEAL N.

GLUTEUS MAXIMUS M.

ISCHIAL
TUBEROSITY

A   SCIATIC N.

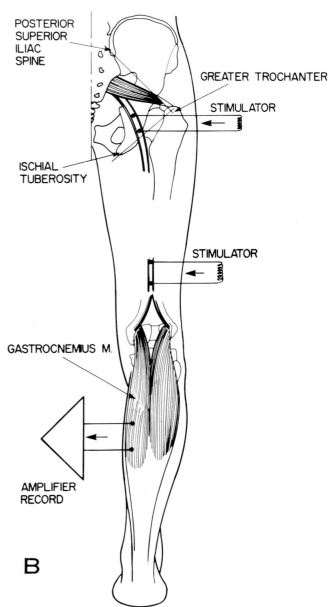

POSTERIOR
SUPERIOR
ILIAC
SPINE

GREATER TROCHANTER

STIMULATOR

ISCHIAL
TUBEROSITY

STIMULATOR

GASTROCNEMIUS M.

AMPLIFIER
RECORD

B

V B 2 Sciatic
(A) Sciatic notch
(B) Electrostimulation

Figure *A* shows the relationship of the sciatic N to the pyriformis muscle and clearly demonstrates that the differentiation of plexus and high sciatic N lesions can be considerably facilitated by electromyographic (EMG) examination—viz., EMG examination of the gluteus maximus, gluteus medius and the tensor fasciae latae M.

In the usual anatomical configuration, the sciatic N is deep to the pyriformis M but in variation the nerve may pass entirely posterior to the muscle, may pierce it as a single trunk or singularly the peroneal portion will penetrate through to the posterior surface. The muscle has been implicated in the compressive neuropathy, the "pyriformis syndrome," when hypertrophy or spasm compresses the sciatic nerve against the notch.

It is repetitive to state but important to note that the short head of the biceps femoris is distinctly innervated from the peroneal rather than the tibial portion of the sciatic!

Figure *B* shows the sites of stimulation in carrying out conduction studies of the sciatic N. Needle electrodes are required. The favored proximal site is at the point of bisection of a line connecting the ischial tuberosity and the greater trochanter. In this location the sciatic N is at a most superficial level. Somewhat more proximally the sciatic may also be stimulated by placement of the electrodes at the point of junction of the middle one-third and lateral two-thirds of a line between the posterosuperior iliac spine and the greater trochanter. The distal stimulation point is at the midline of the apex of the popliteal space. Recording is from the gastrocnemius M (see also "Popliteus M," p. 117).

V B 3   LUMBAR PLEXUS

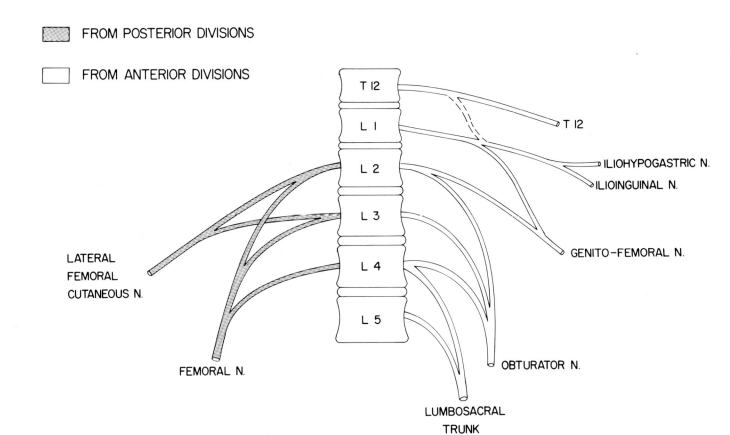

FROM POSTERIOR DIVISIONS

FROM ANTERIOR DIVISIONS

V B 3   Lumbar plexus (diagram)

The plexus is formed from the anterior rami of L_1 to L_4 and usually some fibers from T_{12}. As a parallel to the formation of the brachial plexus, there is a division into anterior and posterior parts which are artifically segregated in the diagram to right and left sides, respectively. The root contributions are more readily identified than in the brachial plexus since the interchanging of nerves is considerably less than in the arm. For example, L_2, L_3 go to the lateral femoral cutaneous N and L_2, L_3, L_4 to the femoral N.

V B 4   OBTURATOR NERVE

V B 5   LATERAL FEMORAL CUTANEOUS

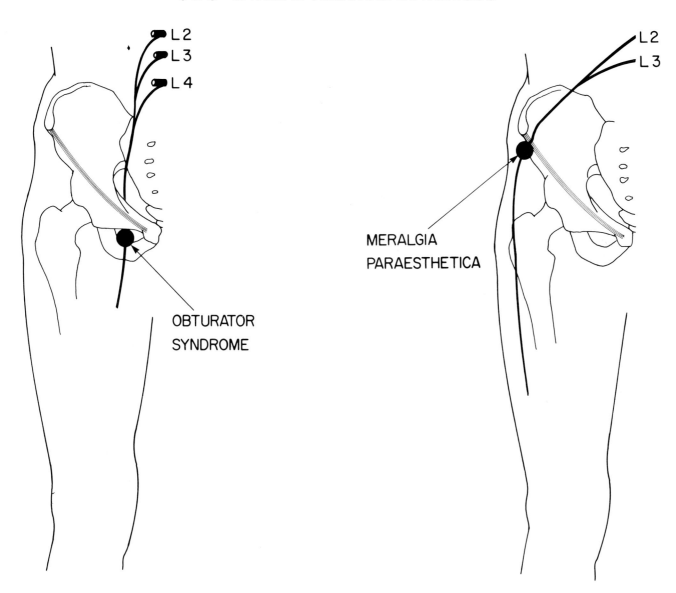

V B 4   Obutrator (diagram)

The obturator N runs a fairly direct course through the obturator foramen to the medial side of the thigh. Aside from direct trauma, a compression of the nerve may occur as it makes its way through the membraneous foramen (i.e., associated with obturator hernia, pelvic tumor). In EMG study of the adductor group it is important to note that the adductor magnus is partially innervated by the sciatic N and that the adductor longus may get its entire nerve supply from the femoral rather than the obturator N.

V B 5   Lateral femoral cutaneous (diagram)

The clinical syndrome which results from entrapment of this nerve is known as meralgia paraesthetica. The compression occurs as the nerve enters the thigh just distal and medial to the anterior superior spine. At this level it also lies just medial to the sartorius muscle. The nerve is purely sensory so that pathology results in various degrees of altered sensibility.

Approximately 10 cm below the anterosuperior spine, the lateral femoral cutaneous N divides into its posterior and anterior divisions. The latter runs down laterally to the level of the knee.

V B 6   FEMORAL NERVE

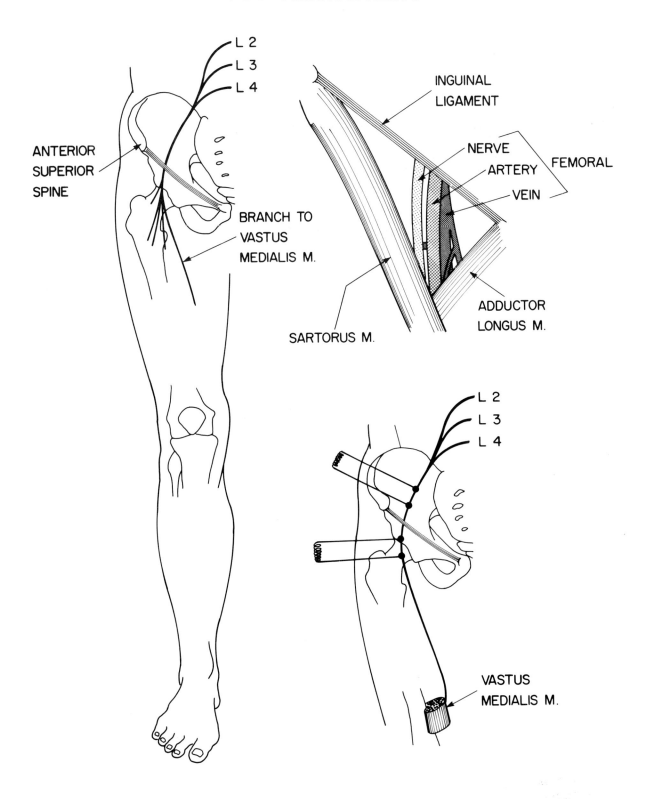

V B 6   Femoral (diagram)

After formation of the nerve trunk, the femoral N goes through the lateral border of the psoas major **M** and passes into the thigh under the inguinal ligament into the femoral triangle. Here it lies on the iliopsoas muscle and is lateral to the femoral artery.

For practical purposes, the branching of the femoral N takes place just below the inguinal ligament with two long branches running distally and medially: (1) the branch supply to the vastus medialis and (2) the saphenous N branch.

V B 7 SAPHENOUS NERVE

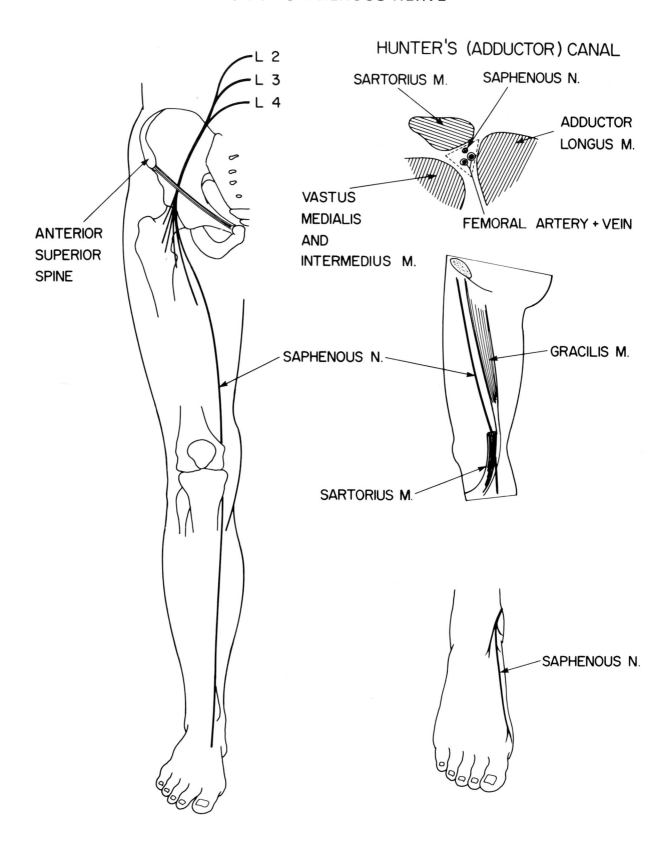

HUNTER'S (ADDUCTOR) CANAL

SARTORIUS M.   SAPHENOUS N.

ADDUCTOR
LONGUS M.

VASTUS
MEDIALIS
AND
INTERMEDIUS M.

FEMORAL ARTERY + VEIN

L 2
L 3
L 4

ANTERIOR
SUPERIOR
SPINE

SAPHENOUS N.

GRACILIS M.

SARTORIUS M.

SAPHENOUS N.

V B 7   Saphenous (diagram)

This branch of the femoral N dips into the adductor canal at the apex of the femoral canal to join the deep femoral vessels. The nerve begins to move to a more superficial position again at the lower end of the adductor canal by passing between the sartorius and adductor magnus M to the medial side of the thigh and then runs down to the medial aspect of the knee where it becomes subcutaneous by passing between the sartorius M and gracilis M. The longest branch of the femoral N then runs a straight course down the leg with the internal saphenous vein to come in front of the medial malleolus and then to the side of the foot to about the metatarsophalangeal joint level.

V B 8 SURAL NERVE

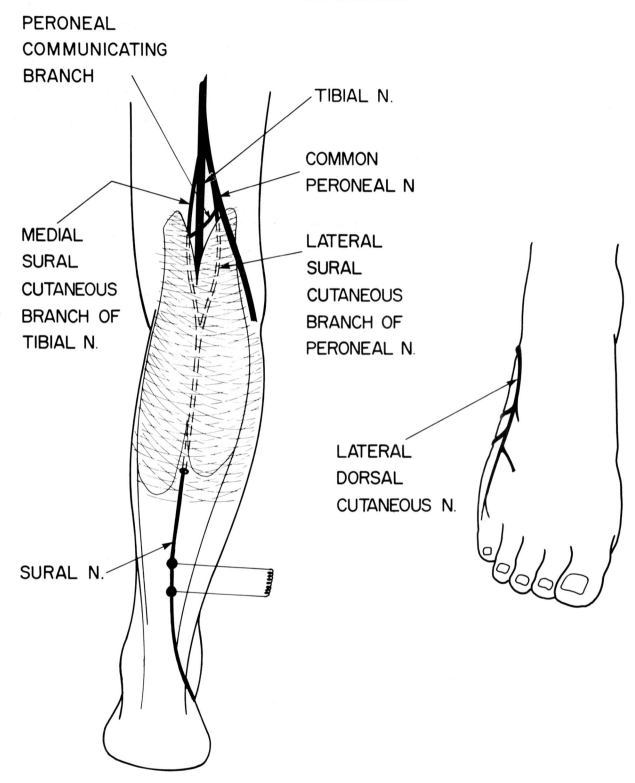

PERONEAL
COMMUNICATING
BRANCH

TIBIAL N.

COMMON
PERONEAL N

MEDIAL
SURAL
CUTANEOUS
BRANCH OF
TIBIAL N.

LATERAL
SURAL
CUTANEOUS
BRANCH OF
PERONEAL N.

SURAL N.

LATERAL
DORSAL
CUTANEOUS N.

V B 8   Sural (diagram)

The sural N is formed from branches derived from the tibial N and peroneal N. The tibial gives rise to the medial sural cutaneous N while in the popliteal space. This is joined by a small twig from the peroneal, the peroneal communicating branch and then by the lateral sural cutaneous branch of the common peroneal. The trunk of the sural which is formed runs down under cover of the deep fascia lying on the gastrocnemius, until mid leg (or at the junction of the upper two-thirds and lower one-third of the leg!). There the deep fascia is pierced and the nerve joins the short (external) saphenous vein to run down behind the lateral malleolus around to the dorsum of the foot, as the lateral dorsal cutaneous N. Anomalies of this descriptive formation of the sural N are not rare.

V B 9   POSTERIOR TIBIAL NERVE

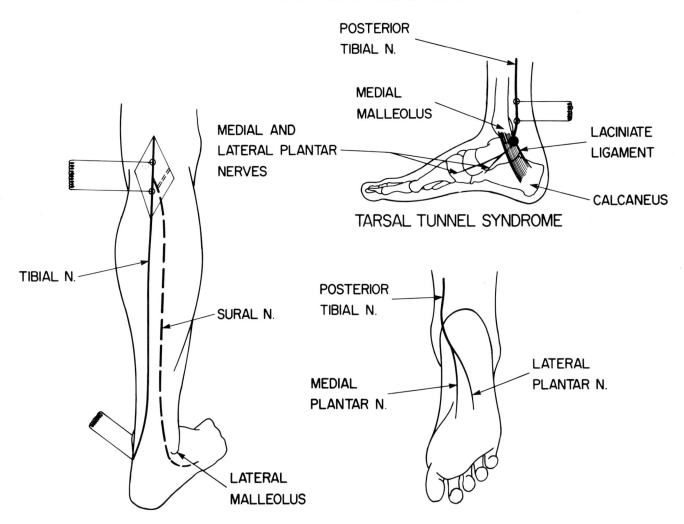

POSTERIOR TIBIAL N.

MEDIAL MALLEOLUS

LACINIATE LIGAMENT

CALCANEUS

MEDIAL AND LATERAL PLANTAR NERVES

TARSAL TUNNEL SYNDROME

TIBIAL N.

SURAL N.

LATERAL MALLEOLUS

POSTERIOR TIBIAL N.

MEDIAL PLANTAR N.

LATERAL PLANTAR N.

V B 9   Posterior tibial (diagram)

The posterior tibial N arises as the medial branch of
the bifurcation of the two portions of the sciatic N at
the upper corner of the quadrangular popliteal space.
The nerve runs down the middle of the space past the
two heads of the gastrocnemius. It then takes a
slightly medial course on a line with the medial
malleolus. It passes inferior to the malleolus through
the tarsal tunnel to enter the foot. At the distal end of
the fibrosseous tunnel it bifurcates into the medial
and lateral plantar N. The muscular and cutaneous
distribution of the medial and lateral plantar N bear a
strong homologous relationship to the median and
ulnar distribution in the hand.

At the proximal end of the tarsal tunnel, the entire
trunk of the posterior tibial N may be compressed to
produce weakness and sensory loss in the medial and
lateral plantar distribution as well as in the distribution of the most proximal sensory branch, the cal-
canean, which supplies the medial surface of the heel.

The evoked muscle action potential of the abductor
hallucis and that of the abductor digiti quinti are
respectively used in motor conduction studies of the
plantar nerves (as well as in tibial nerve conduction
determination).

V B 10 PERONEAL NERVE

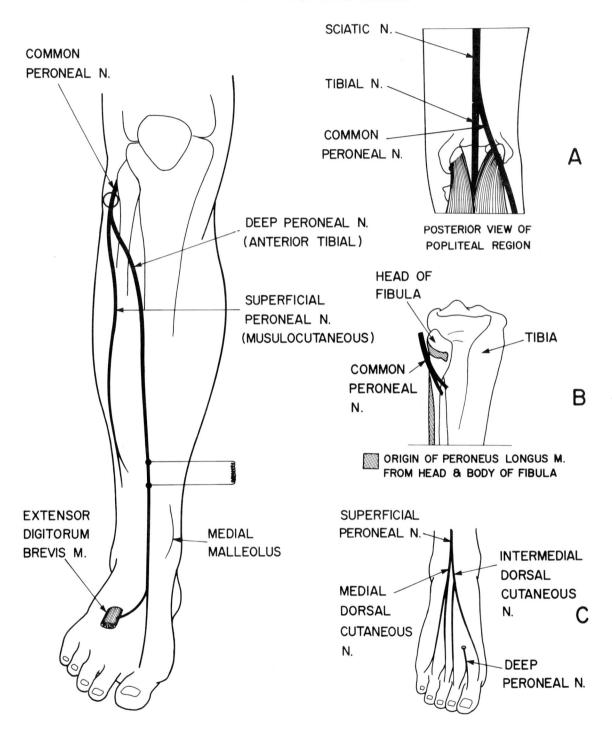

COMMON PERONEAL N.

DEEP PERONEAL N. (ANTERIOR TIBIAL)

SUPERFICIAL PERONEAL N. (MUSULOCUTANEOUS)

EXTENSOR DIGITORUM BREVIS M.

MEDIAL MALLEOLUS

SCIATIC N.

TIBIAL N.

COMMON PERONEAL N.

A

POSTERIOR VIEW OF POPLITEAL REGION

HEAD OF FIBULA

TIBIA

COMMON PERONEAL N.

B

▨ ORIGIN OF PERONEUS LONGUS M. FROM HEAD & BODY OF FIBULA

SUPERFICIAL PERONEAL N.

MEDIAL DORSAL CUTANEOUS N.

INTERMEDIAL DORSAL CUTANEOUS N.

C

DEEP PERONEAL N.

V B 10   Common peroneal (diagram)

The common peroneal N originates from the lateral portion of the sciatic N in the upper part of the popliteal fossa. The nerve moves distally and laterally in line with the tendon of the biceps femoris to the level of the neck of the fibula where it winds around to come into its anterolateral position. The nerve is in juxtaposition to the bone with the origins of the peroneus longus from the head of the fibula (above) and the body of the fibula (below) leaving a slit for the nerve to pass through. At this aperture or just proximal to it, the common peroneal splits into its superficial and deep branches. The superficial peroneal N (musculocutaneous) turns sharply lateral-ward at the edge of the peroneus longus origin to run down to innervate the peroneii and then pierce the fascia to become the cutaneous supply for part of the dorsum of the foot. The deep peroneal N (anterior tibial) moves to a deeper position to ride on the anterior surface of the interosseous membrane where it gives off most of its muscular branches. It then passes under the extensor retinaculum of the ankle and divides into the dorsal medial and lateral nerves of the foot.

V B 11 MEDIAL AND LATERAL PLANTAR NERVES

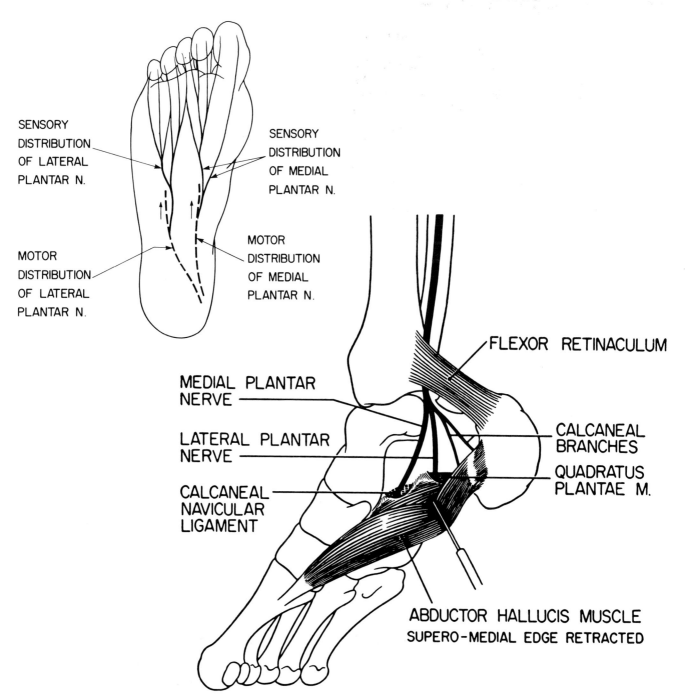

SENSORY DISTRIBUTION OF LATERAL PLANTAR N.

SENSORY DISTRIBUTION OF MEDIAL PLANTAR N.

MOTOR DISTRIBUTION OF LATERAL PLANTAR N.

MOTOR DISTRIBUTION OF MEDIAL PLANTAR N.

FLEXOR RETINACULUM

MEDIAL PLANTAR NERVE

LATERAL PLANTAR NERVE

CALCANEAL BRANCHES

QUADRATUS PLANTAE M.

CALCANEAL NAVICULAR LIGAMENT

ABDUCTOR HALLUCIS MUSCLE
SUPERO-MEDIAL EDGE RETRACTED

V B 11   Medial and lateral plantar (diagram)

The bifurcation of the posterior tibial N into the medial and lateral plantar N takes place in the tarsal tunnel. Beyond the malleolar level the plantar N pass distally through individual apertures in the proximal end of the abductor hallucis M.

Muscle supplied:

Lateral	Medial
Quadratus plantae	Abductor hallucis
Flexor digiti quinti brevis	Flexor hallucis brevis
Adductor hallucis	Flexor digitorum brevis
Lateral lumbricales (3, 4)	Medial lumbricales (1, 2)
Abductor digiti quinti	
Opponens digiti quinti	
Interossei	

Both or either plantar nerves may be injured when still in the tunnel or may be compromised by "entrapment" at the foramina of exit in the abductor hallucis M.

V B 12 CROSS SECTION AT PUBIC TUBERCLE

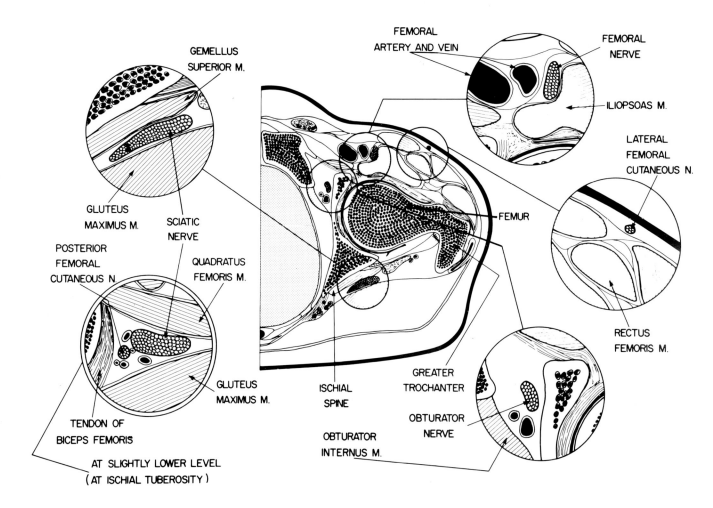

GEMELLUS SUPERIOR M.

FEMORAL ARTERY AND VEIN

FEMORAL NERVE

ILIOPSOAS M.

LATERAL FEMORAL CUTANEOUS N.

GLUTEUS MAXIMUS M.

SCIATIC NERVE

FEMUR

POSTERIOR FEMORAL CUTANEOUS N.

QUADRATUS FEMORIS M.

RECTUS FEMORIS M.

GLUTEUS MAXIMUS M.

TENDON OF BICEPS FEMORIS

ISCHIAL SPINE

GREATER TROCHANTER

OBTURATOR NERVE

OBTURATOR INTERNUS M.

AT SLIGHTLY LOWER LEVEL (AT ISCHIAL TUBEROSITY)

V B 12　Lower extremity nerves
Level: Pubic tubercle cross section

Femoral N—lies in the femoral triangle with the iliopsoas M behind and the femoral artery to its medial side; the femoral vein is of course medial to the artery.

Lateral femoral cutaneous N—is superficial to the fasciae latae having passed through its own tunnel-like passageway. The course of the sartorius muscle is to the medial side of the thigh so that at the pubic tubercle level the lateral femoral cutaneous is lateral to the edge of sartorius M and medial to edge of tensor fasciae latae M.

Sciatic N—is shown at the level of the spine of the ischium where it lies under cover of the gluteus maximus and rests on the gemellus superior M. The position under the gluteus is maintained at the level of the ischial tuberosity but at this point the nerve rests on another of the short muscles, the quadratus femoris.

Obturator N—is seen just as it has passed under the pubic bone. The landmark pubic tubercle is located medially and anteriorly.

V B 13   CROSS SECTION AT MID THIGH

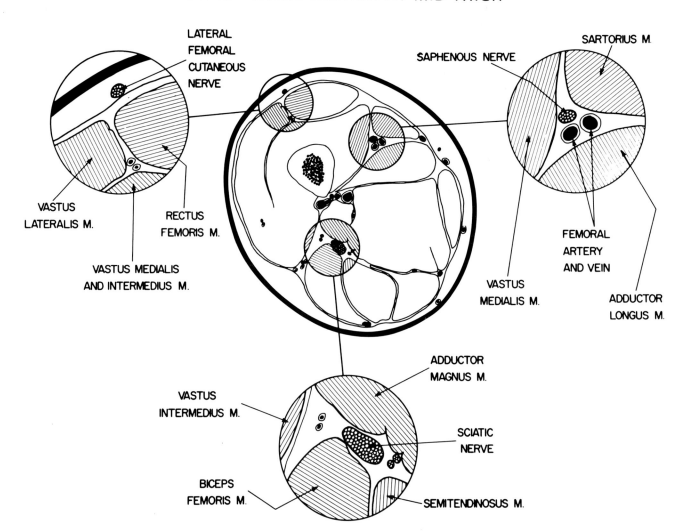

V B 13   Lower extremity nerves
Level: Mid-thigh cross section

Lateral femoral cutaneous N—is now subcutaneous and lies approximately at the lateral edge of the rectus femoris M.

Saphenous N—located in the adductor (Hunter's) canal which is roughly triangular in shape and bound by the sartorius, vastus medialis and adductor longus M.

Sciatic N—runs on the midline of the posterior thigh between the adductor magnus M anteriorly and the hamstring M posteriorly.

V B 14   CROSS SECTION AT PATELLA

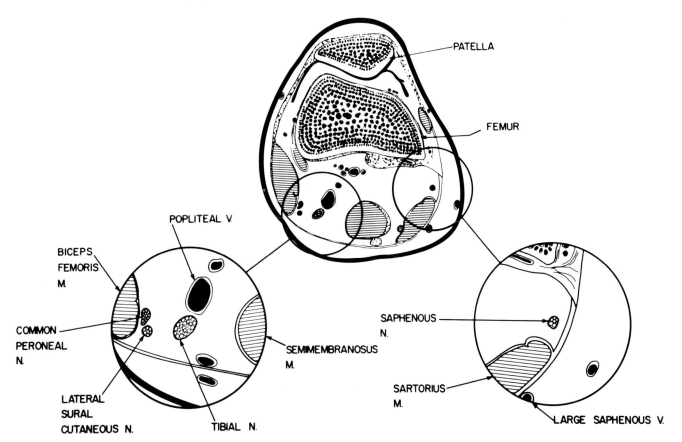

PATELLA

FEMUR

POPLITEAL V

BICEPS
FEMORIS
M.

COMMON
PERONEAL
N.

LATERAL
SURAL
CUTANEOUS N.

TIBIAL N.

SEMIMEMBRANOSUS
M.

SAPHENOUS
N.

SARTORIUS
M.

LARGE SAPHENOUS V.

V B 14   Lower extremity nerves
Level : Cross section through patella

This section runs through the junction of the upper one-third and lower two-thirds of the patella.

Saphenous N. This continuation of the femoral N is internal to the deep fascia and behind the sartorius M. It then moves superficially and laterally between the tendons of the sartorius M and the gracilis M and joins the course of the long saphenous vein.

Common peroneal and posterior tibial N. In this section the tibial N had been displaced a bit from its usual more medial position but the common peroneal is normally situated laterally, adjacent to the tendon of the biceps femoris M. Its cutaneous branch, the lateral sural cutaneous N, is shown in the popliteal space. This branch later joints the medial cutaneous sural N from the posterior tibial N to form the trunk of the sural proper.

V B 15   CROSS SECTION AT HEAD OF FIBULA

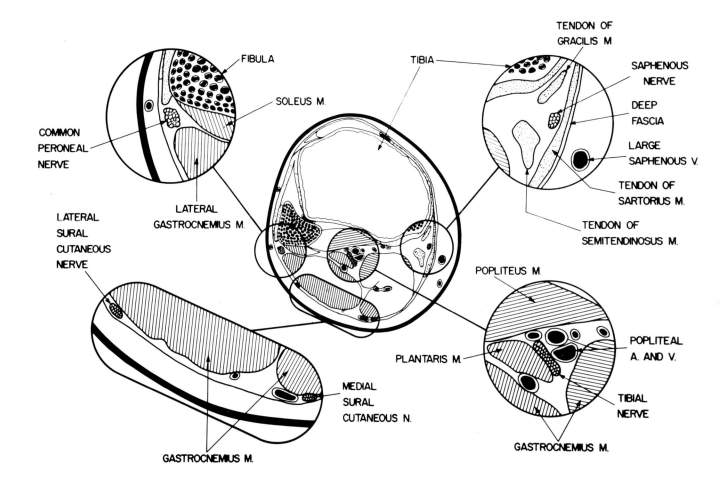

V B 15   Lower extremity nerves
Level: Cross section at head of fibula

Common peroneal N. The main trunk of the nerve has not yet bifurcated and lies at the posterolateral aspect of the head of the fibula adjacent to the edge of the lateral head of the gastrocnemius.

Sural N. The lateral sural cutaneous branch from the common peroneal and the medial sural cutaneous N from the tibial are distinct and lie in position over the gastrocnemius M.

Tibial N—lies just below the margins of the gastrocnemius bellies at the inferior border of the popliteal space. The position of the nerve is deep and in close proximity to the distal part of the popliteus muscle (the floor of the popliteal space) and the popliteal artery and veins.

Saphenous N. The saphenous branch of the femoral N is already medially located between the margins of the tibia and the medial belly of the gastrocnemius but is still internal to the deep fascia of the leg.

V B 16   CROSS SECTION AT MID LEG

EXTENSOR DIGITORUM LONGUS M.

ANTERIOR TIBIALIS M.

DEEP PERONEAL N.

PERONEAL A. AND V.

POSTERIOR TIBIALIS M.

INTEROSSEOUS MEMBRANE

ANTERIOR TIBIALIS A. AND V.

TIBIA

POSTERIOR TIBIALIS A AND V

SUPERFICIAL PERONEAL N.

SAPHENOUS NERVE

TIBIAL NERVE

SOLEUS M

FIBULA

PERONEUS LONGUS AND BREVIS M.

SOLEUS M

GASTROCNEMIUS M.

MEDIAL SURAL CUTANEOUS N.

LATERAL SURAL CUTANEOUS N.

SMALL SAPHENOUS V.

FASCIA

V B 16   Lower extremity nerves
Level: Mid-leg cross section

Saphenous N—is superficial to the deep fascia and runs down the leg with the internal or long saphenous vein.

Sural N. The combined trunk of the sural has not yet been formed from its lateral and medial contributors although it frequently does so at this level of the leg. The other common site where medial and lateral sural cutaneous N join is at the junction of lower one-third with upper two-thirds of the leg.

Peroneal N. The deep peroneal (anterior tibial) is anterior to the interosseous membrane under cover of the anterior tibial M and extensor digitorum longus M. The superficial peroneal descends with the peroneal muscles in the lateral compartment of the leg. This nerve is not subcutaneous but is close to the fibula.

Post tibial N—lies deep in the leg on the anterior surface of the soleus M and posterior to the posterior tibial N.

V B 17   CROSS SECTION APPROX. 10 cm ABOVE LATERAL MALLEOLUS

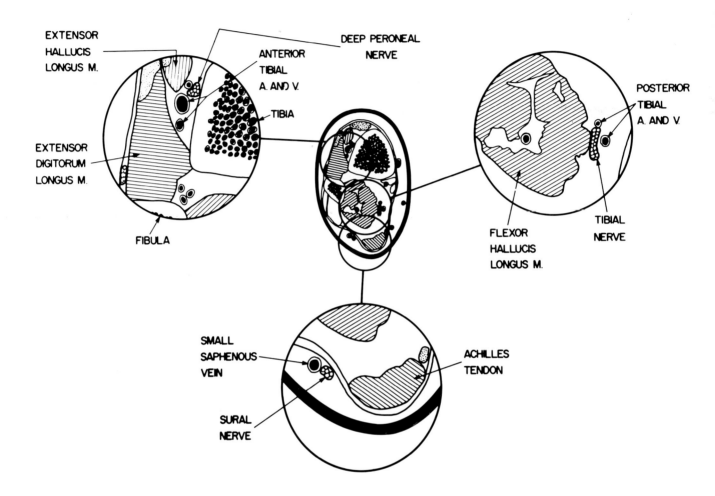

V B 17   Lower extremity nerves
Level: Cross section about 10 cm above lateral malleolus

Anterior tibial N (deep peroneal). This level is above the superior extensor retinaculum of the leg. The nerve runs with the artery and vein close to the lateral margin of the tibia and is best identified by its close proximity to the extensor hallucis longus M and tendon.

Posterior tibial N—is in a posterior position on a line with the posterior aspect of the medial malleolus and the easily palpated posterior tibial artery. At the upper margin of the malleolus, the nerve is close to the posterolateral margin of the bone.

Sural N—is located on the opposite aspect of the leg with respect to the malleolus; it runs parallel to the lateral edge of the achilles tendon.

V B 18   CROSS SECTION AT FOREFOOT

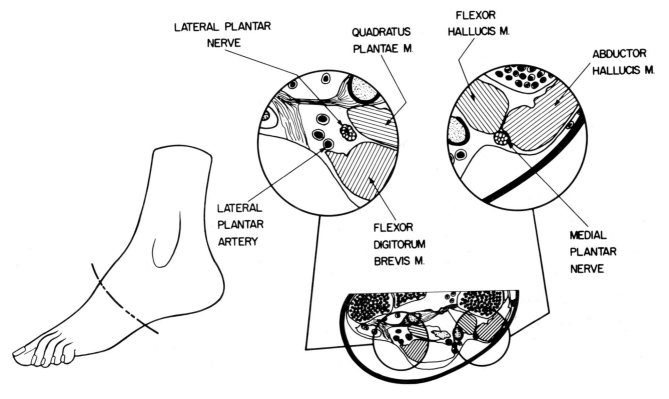

LATERAL PLANTAR
NERVE

QUADRATUS
PLANTAE M.

FLEXOR
HALLUCIS M.

ABDUCTOR
HALLUCIS M.

LATERAL
PLANTAR
ARTERY

FLEXOR
DIGITORUM
BREVIS M.

MEDIAL
PLANTAR
NERVE

V B 18   Lower extremity nerves
Level: Cross section at forefoot

The main trunks of the lateral and medial plantar N are quite close to the plantar fascia at this level. The medial lies in close proximity to the abductor hallucis M, whereas the lateral lies on the quadratus plantae adjacent to the edge of the flexor digitorum brevis. The lateral plantar N runs in a direction toward the base of the fifth metatarsal bone.

INDEX

Anterior interosseous syndrome, 69
Arcade of Frohse, 73

Carpal tunnel, 62, 89
Cervical rib, 71
Cross sections, lower extremity, at
  forefoot, 151
  head of fibula, 148
  malleolus (10 cm above), 150
  mid leg, 149
  mid thigh, 146
  patella, 147
  pubic tubercle, 145
Cross sections, upper extremity, at
  distal carpal bones, 89
  epicondyles, 83
  forearm, above radial styloid
    5 cm above, 79
    9 cm above, 77
    12 cm above, 77
  forearm, below epicondyle (7.5 cm), 75
  mid arm, 81
  mid forearm, 85
  radial styloid, 87
Cubital tunnel, 71

Femoral triangle, 132

Guyon's canal, 71, 89

Hunter's canal, 134

Ligament of Struthers, 65

Meralgia paraesthetica, 131
Muscles
  abdominal, 97
  abductor digiti quinti (hand), 53
  abductor digiti quinti (foot), 121
  abductor hallucis, 121
  abductor pollicis brevis, 51
  abductor pollicis longus, 49
  adductor longus, 113
  anconeus, 35
  auricular posterior, 5
  biceps brachii, 33
  biceps femoris (short head), 111
  brachialis, 33
  brachioradialis, 36
  coracobrachialis, 31
  deltoid, 28
  extensor digitorum brevis, 123
  extensor digitorum longus, 115
  extensor hallucis longus, 116
  extensor indicis proprius, 49
  external oblique (abdominal), 97
  facial (expression), 3
  first dorsal interosseous, 53
  flexor carpi radialis, 36
  flexor carpi ulnaris, 38
  flexor digitorum brevis, 121

flexor digitorum profundus, 39
flexor digitorum sublimis, 39
flexor pollicis brevis, 51
flexor pollicis longus, 40
frontalis, 3
gastrocnemius, 119
gluteus maximus, 109
gluteus medius, 109
hamstrings, 113
iliopsoas, 102
infraspinatus, 17
intercostals, 25
latissimus dorsi, 23
levator scapulae, 7
lumbricales, 55
masseter, 3
mentalis, 3
multifidus, 95
opponens pollicis, 51
orbicularis oculi, 3
orbicularis oris, 3
paraspinal (cervical), 11
paraspinal (lumbar), 95
pectoralis (major and minor), 21
peroneus brevis, 115
peroneus longus, 115
popliteus, 117
pronator quadratus, 41, 68
pronator teres, 37, 66
quadriceps femoris, 113
rectus abdominis, 97
rhomboid major, 15
rhomboid minor, 15
sartorius, 113
serratus anterior, 18
soleus, 119
sphincter ani, 99
sternocleidomastoid, 9
supinator, 47
supraspinatus, 17
tensor fasciae latae, 107
tibialis anterior, 115
tibialis posterior, 125
tongue, 7
trapezius, 15
triceps brachii, 34
triceps surae, 119

Nerves
  anterior interosseous, 41, 66, 69
  anterior thoracic (medial and lateral), 21
  anterior tibial (deep peroneal), 115
  axillary, 28
  brachial plexus, 57, 59, 61
  coccygeal plexus, 126
  digital (hand), 91
  dorsal scapular, 9, 15
  facial, 3
    posterior auricular branch, 5
  femoral, 113, 133
  hypoglossal, 7

iliohypogastric, 97, 130
ilioinguinal, 97, 130
inferior gluteal, 109
inferior hemorrhoidal (branch of pudendal), 99
lateral femoral cutaneous, 131
lateral plantar, 121, 143
long thoracic, 18
lumbar plexus, 130
medial plantar, 121, 143
median, 36, 37, 39–41, 51, 55, 63, 66
musculocutaneous, 31, 33
obturator, 113, 131
peroneal, common, 141
  deep branch, 115, 116, 123
  superficial branch (musculocutane-
    ous), 115
posterior interosseous, 49
posterior tibial, 125, 139
pudendal, 98, 99, 126
radial, 33–36, 73
  superficial and deep branches, 47, 77,
    79
sacral plexus, 126, 127
saphenous, 135
sciatic, 111, 113, 129
spinal accessory, 9, 15
superior gluteal, 107, 109
suprascapular, 17
sural, 137
temporal (deep anterior and posterior),
  93
thoracodorsal, 23
tibial, 117, 119
trigeminal, 3
ulnar, 38, 39, 51, 53, 55, 71
Neurovascular bundle (intercostal), 25

Obturator syndrome, 131

Pneumothorax, 18, 25
Posterior interosseous syndrome, 67, 72
Pyriformis syndrome, 129

Saturday night palsy, 72
Supinator syndrome, 72, 73
Syndromes
  anterior interosseous, 62, 68
  carpal tunnel, 62, 89
  obturator, 131
  posterior interosseous, 67, 72
  pronator, 62, 67
  pyriformis, 129
  supinator, 72, 73
  tarsal tunnel, 138
  thoracic outlet, 71
  ulnar tunnel, 71, 89

Tarsal tunnel, 138
Thoracic outlet, 71

Ulnar tunnel (canal of Guyon), 71